A Homoeopathic Approach to Cancer

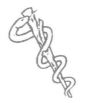

OTHER BOOKS BY CATHERINE R. COULTER

Portraits of Homœopathic Medicines
Psychophysical Analyses of Selected Constitutional Types
Vol. 1: ISBN 978-0971308213 (0971308217)
Vol. 2: ISBN 978-0971308220 (0971308225)

Expanding Views of the Materia Medica
(includes "Portrait of Indifference")
Vol. 3: ISBN 978-0971308237 (0971308233)

Nature and Human Personality: Homœopathic Archetypes
ISBN 978-0971308244 (0971308241)

Homœopathic Sketches of Children's Types
ISBN 978-0971308268 (0971308268)

Homœopathic Education: The Unfolding of Experience
ISBN 978-0971308275

GERMAN
Krebs–Ein homöopathischer Behandlungsansatz
Translated by Ulrike Kessler
ISBN 978-0971308251 (097130825X)

FRENCH
Archétypes Homéopathiques
Translated by Alexa deBournand
ISBN 978-0971308282 (0971308284)

✦

All books are available from:

Ninth House Publishing
260 J R Hawvermale Way
Berkeley Springs WV 25411
Telephone: 1-800-336-1695 • www.homeopathyworks.com

A HOMOEOPATHIC APPROACH TO CANCER

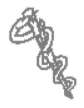

Dr. A.U. Ramakrishnan

M.B.B.S., M.F. Hom. [London]

and

Catherine R. Coulter

NINTH HOUSE PUBLISHING
Berkeley Spring, West Virginia

This book presents current scientific information and opinion pertinent to medical and homoeopathic professionals. It does not provide advice concerning specific diagnosis and treatment of individual cases and is not intended for use by the layperson. The authors and publisher will not be responsible or liable for actions taken as a result of the opinions expressed in this book.

EDITORS   Marian Coulter
          Mary Yano
          Suzanne Wakefield

PRODUCTION   Barbara Shaw

COVER DESIGN   Diane Beasley

Printed in the United States of America
by McNaughton & Gunn, Inc.

Ninth House Publishing
260 J R Hawvermale Way
Berkeley Springs, West Virginia 25411
Telephone: 1-800-336-1695
Web site: www.homeopathyworks.com

LIBRARY OF CONGRESS CATALOGING-IN-PUBLICATION DATA

Ramakrishnan, A.U.
    A Homoeopathic Approach to Cancer / by A.U. Ramakrishnan and
    Catherine R. Coulter.
        p. 272; 24 cm.
    Includes bibliographical references and index.
    ISBN 0-9713082-0-9
    1. Cancer—Homeopathic treatment. I. Coulter, Catherine R. II. Title.
    [DNLM: 1. Homeopathy—methods. 2. Neoplasms—therapy. QZ 266 R165h
    2001]
RX261.C3 R35 2001
616.99'406—dc21

2001019433

To my beloved father

Dr. A. Umapathi Mudaliar
M.B.B.S., M.F. Hom. [London]

whose life and breath was homoeopathy.
He is the one who taught me, trained me, and
is responsible for whatever good there is in me, and
to whom I owe my life and soul.

✦

A.U. Ramakrishnan

Acknowledgments

A particular debt of gratitude is owed to two people: first and foremost to Eileen Isison, without whose initiative this book might never have been written. She not only introduced the two authors but was also ever willing to be consulted on matters related to cancer and to assist with her substantial knowledge of the subject.

The second person is Mary Yano. Her thoughtful suggestions and tireless support throughout the typing of this manuscript lie beyond any ordinary thanks or acknowledgments.

One other person deserves special mention: Betty Wood, M.D., for her careful reading of and comments on the text.

Contents

Introduction

Dr. A.U. Ramakrishnan

For more than thirty years I have been practicing homoeopathy and lecturing on the subject. Recently I have felt that I should put down my thoughts in book form and thus have a chance to share my experience with others, who then could also profit from the homoeopathic healing method.

I was trained in allopathic medicine in India, at the prestigious Madras Medical College and graduated in 1966. Then I went to England and was trained in homoeopathy, under the particular tutelage of Dr. Margery G. Blackie, at the Royal London Homoeopathic Hospital, and got my M.F. Hom. in 1968. Since then I have been teaching and conducting postgraduate courses in India, East Asia, Western Europe, and North America, and have been offering consultations to patients all over the world.

What led me to focus on cancer was a series of failures in cancer cases in my earlier days, particularly the loss of my sister in 1974 and my elder brother in 1984, both of whom were homoeopathic doctors. From that time on I have been trying out different combinations, potencies, and dosages of remedies in the treatment of this disease.

Beginning in the late 1980s, I began to observe favorable responses and over the next few years embarked on and experimented with a new technique of prescribing. This methodology, which I have named my

"Plussing Method," stabilized around 1993. The good results of the seven years or so of working very intensely with this method, especially in comparison with my work in cancer of the previous years, gave me a sense of happiness and enthusiasm that prompted me to write a book.

At this juncture I was fortunate to meet Catherine R. Coulter, the well-known writer on homoeopathic *materia medica,* with whom I found a lot of agreement in our thoughts on homoeopathic theory and practice and, hence, decided to write this book with her. She has contributed to this work her profound knowledge and understanding of homoeopathy and her forty years experience of teaching, lecturing, and training physicians by the preceptorship method.

I would also like to express my appreciation of the efforts of a very dear friend of mine, Eileen Isison. She has helped me right from the beginning by coordinating my work, encouraging me when my spirits flagged, and helping me to realize the dream of bringing out this book, *A Homoeopathic Approach to Cancer.*

Dr. A.U. Ramakrishnan

Honorary Homoeopathic Physician to the President of India
Formerly:
    President, Homoeopathic Medical Association of India, Tamil Nadu State Branch
    Honorary Advisor to the Government of Tamil Nadu
    Member, Scientific Advisory Board, CCRIMH, Government of India, New Delhi
    Member, Board of Examiners for DHMS Course, Government of Tamil Nadu
    Member, Governing Body of National Institute of Homoeopathy, Calcutta
    Member, Homoeopathic Pharmacopoeia Committee, Government of India
    Member, Board of Studies, Madurai Kamaraj University, Tamil Nadu
    Chairman, Board of Studies, Dr. M.G.R. Medical University, Madras
    Member, Central Council of Homoeopathy, Government of India
    Member, Scientific Advisory Committee, CCRH, New Delhi

Introduction

Catherine R. Coulter

It has been an extremely rewarding experience for me to author this book on Dr. Ramakrishnan's method. During the course of close to four decades of teaching and training physicians, I have always been looking for ways to transmit homoeopathic knowledge and experience, and this unprecedented volume of cases of one type of disease in all its variations offered two distinct opportunities. First, every prescribing point raised, subtle as well as significant, could be illustrated and substantiated by one or more case examples; and second, the several thousand cancer cases treated by Dr. Ramakrishnan constituted a critical mass of data that allowed patterns to emerge—patterns of symptoms and patterns of prescribing—which are crucial to recognize in the treatment of the different stages of this complex disease.

The principal challenge in presenting the large number of cases in this book was not only how to select, organize, and interpret them, but, above all, how to devise a clear, concise yet comprehensive format which would convey Dr. Ramakrishnan's invaluable knowledge in such a way as to be usable by practitioners less experienced than himself. For Dr. Ramakrishnan's expertise stems, in part, from a background uniquely steeped in a rich national, cultural, and family tradition of homoeopathy. Indeed, for one physician to have the opportunity to treat personally, by the homoeopathic method, more than 5,000 cancer cases necessitated a doctor from India—the only country in the world in which homoeopathy enjoys tremendous prestige and in which an estimated ten million of its population use homoeopathy routinely for even the most severe diseases.

Naturally, there arises the question of the need for familiarity with the homoeopathic philosophy and methodology. Certainly, the more experienced in this discipline the prescriber, the easier it is for him or her to master the Ramakrishnan Method—and the better will be the results. And the procedural analyses and observations on methodology interspersed throughout the text should help guide the committed practitioner to correct prescribing. Be it noted, however, that because the remarks on the treatment of one type of cancer often apply to another, the book ought to be read in its entirety before commencing treatment by the Ramakrishnan Method. It is not sufficient to peruse only those pages dealing with the particular type of cancer under current treatment.

Finally, it is my hope that the information and material presented in this volume will be instructive to many types of doctors and practitioners—and will encourage those who have studied and been practicing the science to employ homoeopathy in conjunction with their own particular medical disciplines and healing methods.

Catherine R. Coulter, M.A.
Honorary Life Member of the American Institute of Homeopathy

ADVISORY NOTE

This book is not a self-help manual.
The information in it should be applied only under
the direction of a knowledgeable homoeopathic practitioner
or a doctor or alternative therapist using homoeopathy in
conjunction with his or her particular discipline.

Chapter 1
The Homoeopathic Approach

Treatment of the Individual

The science of homoeopathy, founded by Samuel Hahnemann around the beginning of the nineteenth century, is based on the Law of Similars. This means that a medicinal substance capable of producing a set of morbid symptoms in the healthy individual will remove similar symptoms occurring in an individual suffering from illness. From this basic tenet there evolves a strict set of rules that governs the administration of its medicines.* But homoeopathy is so vast and multifaceted in its healing action that it encompasses a number of distinct approaches in its methodology. Not only does every practitioner have a particular style, but the illnesses themselves are approached by different methods.

In the strictest classical tradition, the way to prescribe is to administer a single dose of a single remedy (the one that corresponds most closely or is the most "similar" to a patient's totality of symptoms)—then wait and observe what changes the remedy has or has not accomplished before proceeding to the next dose (or to the next appropriate remedy when the first remedy ceases to act). Carrying this sparing and highly individualized approach to illness a step further, homoeopathy arrives at the concept of the "constitutional remedy." This term signifies the medicinal substance that encompasses not only the sum total of a patient's physical, mental,

---

*It does not lie within the parameters of this book to present a thorough and detailed treatise on the philosophy, principles, and practices of the homoeopathic discipline. The reader unfamiliar with these is urged to consult any one of a number of books available on the subject.

1

and emotional symptoms, but his personality picture as well. To take, for instance, a *Phosphorus* patient: generally he (or she) will be of slender build, with small, regular features and arresting eyes, and will display an attractive, friendly manner. There is a strong desire for cold drinks and a liking for both salt and foods with a zesty flavor. The type is susceptible to affections of the throat, chest, bones, and blood. The personality is bright, sensitive, impressionable, affectionate, highly responsive to another's wavelength—with a love for excitement, romance, and artistic pursuits; but also likely to harbor many fears: of being abandoned, of illness, of thunderstorms—or merely free-floating anxieties. Thus, in prescribing "constitutionally," the homoeopathic practitioner must be sensitive not only to the modalities and subtle differentiations of the symptoms, but to the shadings and nuances of personality as well.*

Treatment of the Specific Disease

However, in acute ailments and highly specific types of illnesses (such as cases of poison ivy, chickenpox, high fevers, or influenza), a limited number of medicines appear to work best, regardless of personality type. These are called "specific remedies," in that they address the specific disease itself rather than the patient's complex of physical, mental, and emotional symptoms. So it is in the treatment of cancer. Because of the severity and in many cases urgency of this condition, the individuality of the patient must yield to the "specificity" of the disease itself. Furthermore, with this disease, one is dealing with a measurable pathology and not with subtle imbalances of the body's energies, and therefore less subtle methods of prescribing are required. The very *concreteness* of the tumor, combined as it so often is with a race against time, calls for a more specialized (as against individualized) mode of prescribing.

---

*The subject of constitutional prescribing in cancer cases is dealt with in detail in Chapter 7.

Dr. Ramakrishnan's Method Defined

As mentioned above, in classical homoeopathy the traditional way of prescribing is to administer only one remedy at a time and on an infrequent basis. (To be sure, in acute conditions or where there is pain, severe discomfort, or danger, the remedy may be repeated more frequently, but this is decided according to a patient's manifest individual needs.) In the treatment of cancer, however, the prescriber often cannot afford to "Wait and Watch"; the adverse effects of primary and secondary lesions require a more aggressive procedure. Adapting to the urgency and severity of the condition and to the necessity of quickly bringing about tangible or visible changes in the pathology, Dr. Ramakrishnan has developed a method that involves:

1. *More frequent administrations of a remedy* on a regulated (not "as-needed") basis.

2. *Prescribing a second remedy in alternation with the first,* on a regular (usually weekly) basis *(as described in Chapter 2).* The justification for this last is threefold: (a) a patient's body can tire of a remedy and after a while cease to respond to it; (b) too frequent repetition of a single remedy can cause aggravations (these risks are obviated by the alternating method); (c) addressing the disease on two different levels constitutes a stronger method of attack.

3. *Administering a remedy by the Plussing Method.* This procedure, which has its roots in Hahnemann's discussion of the fifty-millesimal (LM) potencies*—and which was followed by Hahnemann's early disciples, then passed on to homoeopaths worldwide—boasts a number of variations. But essentially it involves diluting a given remedy in water and taking a spoonful of it at regular intervals, stirring before every dose (this last is done in order slightly to change the potency or vibration of the medicine). Plussing not only minimizes further the risk of aggravation but also ensures a medicine's more powerful impact.

Organon of Medicine, paragraphs 247, 248, 272, and elsewhere (see Bibliography of Works Cited).

Dr. Ramakrishnan's particular Plussing Method *consists of diluting three pellets or globules of the remedy (or a number of grains or granules amounting to the size of a pea) in eleven teaspoons of spring water.* * *The patient sips one teaspoon every fifteen minutes. Between each dose, the water is gently stirred or, if in a bottle, shaken once. The patient takes ten teaspoonfuls over the course of approximately two and a half hours and reserves the last teaspoon for the next day. The next day ten teaspoons of fresh water are added to the original mixture (but not any fresh medicine) and the process is repeated. The procedure continues for seven days—after which the remedy is changed and the same procedure is repeated with the new medicine. In weeks 3 and 4 (and every subsequent week), the patient starts with a mixture of fresh water and fresh medicine.*

4. Additionally (and once again, for stronger impact), Dr. Ramakrishnan often employs a Split Dose Method when prescribing single doses of a given remedy. Here, a remedy is taken four times during the course of a day, according to the patient's convenience (typically, the first dose is taken in the early morning, the second before noon, the third sometime during the afternoon, and the fourth before bedtime). This procedure, usually followed *for one day only* (whether one day a week, one day every two weeks, one day every month, or every few months) once the cancer has healed or is under control, generally involves a regular alternation of two remedies—and will henceforth be indicated by the expression "alternating monthly (weekly)."

In the following pages we will examine, largely by means of case examples, this more specialized Ramakrishnan Method, including the most appropriate homoeopathic remedies for different types of cancer and the most effective way of prescribing them—both for the relief of pain and discomfort and during the process of healing.

---

*For more on the size of a "dose" of a remedy, see Appendix, Question 14.

Chapter 2
Principal Remedies
Used for Cancer

Fortunately for the homoeopath confronted with the formidable task of prescribing for cancer, there exists a small number of "cancer" remedies of tried and proven effectiveness.* These can be divided into three groups: the cancer nosodes, the wide-spectrum cancer specifics, and the organ-specific remedies.

The Cancer Nosodes

The homoeopathic nosodes (or medicines made of potentized extractions of diseased matter) are traditionally regarded as cutting deeper than most of the other remedies, in that they are able to affect a patient's inherited susceptibility or predisposition to specific diseases. The homoeopathic method being based on the Law of Similars, it follows that the two sovereign remedies in the treatment of cancer are those prepared from cancer cells. One or the other will be needed in virtually every case.

---

*In presenting the *materia medica,* the authors have judged it most expedient to concentrate on the more specific "cancer remedies"—rather than offer description of the better-known and more widely used medicines, such as *Sulphur, Calcarea carbonica, Natrum muriaticum, Silica, Medorrhinum,* and others. Even though these polychrests (as they are called) are regularly employed when treating cancer, they will only be described insofar as they relate to specific cases.

The most frequently used remedy is *Carcinosin,* prepared from the diseased tissue of a cancer of the breast (and sometimes, depending on the different manufacturers, with added cells from some other types of cancer, such as lung). The British doctors J. Compton Burnett and John Henry Clarke were among the earliest homoeopaths to treat cancer with *Carcinosin.* To Dr. Donald Foubister's clinical experience with children, homoeopathy is indebted for a fuller understanding of the remedy. And Dr. Ramakrishnan, with his extensive treatment of cancer with *Carcinosin,* has carried our appreciation of the remedy's extraordinary healing powers still further. Most notably, this is the preferred nosode when there is a family history of cancer.

The second nosode, *Scirrhinum,* is prepared from a cancer of the liver. As was established by Dr. Margery Blackie and others before her, this remedy is used in preference to *Carcinosin* when the affected gland, lump, or tumor is *stony hard*—especially in cancers of the *breast, lungs, liver, rectum, and prostate,* and sometimes in cancers of the uterus (as in Cases 51 and 52) or leukemia (as in Cases 60 and 61). One can also switch to *Scirrhinum* if the patient is not responding sufficiently well to *Carcinosin* or if, during the course of treatment, the tumor or affected organ becomes hard or the liver is affected. By the same token, one can switch to *Carcinosin* when *Scirrhinum* is not working sufficiently well (see Case 76) or one can alternate back and forth between the two (see Cases 40 and 67). These two cancer remedies, remarkably versatile in action, are prescribed:

1. Alternately with an organ-specific or constitutional remedy to combat and heal the existing cancer;

2. To prevent relapses and recurrences;

3. As palliative remedies in the more advanced stages of the disease, together with other palliative medicines *(see Chapters 5 and 6);* and

4. As prevention when there is a family history of cancer or in precancerous conditions *(see Chapter 9).*

The Wide-Spectrum Cancer Specifics

Other remedies that figure prominently in a large number of cancer cases are *Conium, Thuja,* and *Arsenicum album.*

1. Like *Scirrhinum, Conium* presents the picture of a *stony hard* tumor or gland and has proven of inestimable value in cancers of the *oesophagus, breast, stomach, liver, and prostate.* In this last, if the prostate-specific antigen (PSA) count is high (above 7), then *Conium* plays the role of a specific organ remedy. It also plays an important role in cancer metastasized to the bones.

2. *Thuja,* a remedy that displays the picture of a variety of fungoid and skin growths (including warts, moles, tabs, cauliflower excrescences, etc.), has likewise proven to be of great benefit in cancerous growths—particularly those of the *stomach, colon, rectum, bladder, ovaries, uterus,* and, once again, *prostate,* when the PSA count is moderately high (between 4 and 7).

3. The importance of *Arsenicum album* in the treatment of cancer is indicated in Boericke's *Repertory and Materia Medica,* where, in his introduction to the remedy, the author states that *Arsenicum album* "maintains the system under the stress of malignancy *regardless of location*" (emphasis added). Indeed, apart from its healing properties during the earlier stages, the majority of advanced cases of cancer under systematic homoeopathic treatment will, at some point, require *Arsenicum album* for relief of pain or discomfort, especially during the terminal stage *(see Chapter 6).*

The Organ-Specific Remedies

Through clinical experience and the homoeopathic provings,* it has been ascertained that certain remedies have a strong affinity with some particular organ or with the site of the primary tumor. These have been

---

*Provings are a method of ascertaining the curative properties of the homoeopathic remedies by means of administering small doses of a medicinal substance to healthy human beings and then observing and recording the symptoms elicited by this procedure.

successfully employed in their "specific" roles. Listed in alphabetical order, they are:

ALOE FOR CANCER OF THE COLON AND RECTUM. Symptoms pointing to this remedy are: bleeding from rectum and/or blood in stool; stool jelly-like or mixed with mucus, which is at times bloodstained; cutting or burning pains. Heavy pressure and bloated feeling in abdomen—often from flatus; but patient is uncertain whether flatus or stool will pass. Worse in early morning, from heat; better from cool air.

See Cases 38 and 41.

ARSENICUM BROMATUM AND ARSENICUM IODATUM FOR SKIN CANCER AND SKIN INFECTIONS. Generally speaking, *Arsenicum bromatum* is used for squamous and basal cell carcinomas, melanomas, radiation effects on the skin, and when there are symptoms of intense redness or burning, ulceration, but no infection. *Arsenicum iodatum* is employed for skin lesions that are infected, resulting in sloughing, necrosis at or around the site of the tumor—also when the skin infection has become systemic, with alteration in total white blood count, differential count, and erythrocyte sedimentation rate (ESR). Additionally, *Arsenicum iodatum* can be prescribed in conjunction with other cancer remedies in infections of the urinary tract, for abscesses, a badly infected lung, etc. In these cases, the preferred potency is 6x given several times a day for several weeks.

See Case 68 for *Arsenicum bromatum* and Cases 5, 64, 70, 104, 118, and 119 for *Arsenicum iodatum*.

AURUM MURIATICUM FOR CANCER OF THE ORAL CAVITY. This is the preferred remedy for cancerous ulcers in the inner aspect of the cheeks or on the tongue and palate. Ulcers have everted edges, an indurated base, with submandibular/cervical adenitis; there also may be excessive salivation and a foul odor.

See Cases 5, 13, 14, 15, and 122.

AURUM MURIATICUM NATRONATUM FOR CANCER OF THE UTERUS, OVARIES, AND CERVIX. The principal symptoms of this remedy are ulcerations and induration. There can also be prolapse, leucorrhea, ovarian dropsy, and ossified uterus.

See Cases 3, 52, 87, 88, 119, 120, and 125.

BARYTA CARBONICA AND BARYTA IODATA FOR CANCER OF THE BRAIN AND LYMPH GLANDS. *Baryta carbonica* has an affinity with tumors of the brain cells: gliomas, astrocytomas, angiomas, etc. *Baryta iodata* has more of an affinity with the endocrine glands, the lymph glands, and the tonsilar area (such as cancer of the pharynx).

See Cases 9 and 12 for *Baryta carbonica* and Case 35 for *Baryta iodata*.

CADMIUM SULPHURATUM FOR CANCER OF THE STOMACH AND PANCREAS. The principal symptom of this remedy is vomiting of black coffee-ground-like matter. Other symptoms are bleeding in the stomach; a cutting, twisting, burning type of pain; and intense chilliness and weakness.

See Cases 80, 93, 102, and 117.

CEANOTHUS AMERICANUS FOR CANCER OF THE SPLEEN, PANCREAS, AND LIVER—ALSO LEUKEMIA. Prominent symptoms of this remedy are spleen enlargement and pain that is worse when lying on the left side, and from motion.

See Cases 62, 81, and 115.

CHELIDONIUM FOR CANCER OF THE LIVER AND GALL BLADDER—BOTH PRIMARY AND SECONDARY DEPOSITS. Pain worse when lying on the right side. Nausea, with or without vomiting, better by eating small amounts of food or from hot water; highly colored urine and clay-colored stool. This remedy can also be taken in tincture form for symptom relief, in conjunction with other cancer remedies, as follows: 6 drops in ½ oz. of water, several times a day or whenever needed.

See Cases 36, 79, 81, 82, 83, and 93.

HEKLA LAVA AND *SYMPHYTUM* FOR BONE AND BLOOD CANCERS. *Hekla lava* is the principal remedy for cancers (both primary and secondary) of the bones: sarcomas, osteoclastomas, myelomas, Ewing's sarcomas, and of other bony growths. It is also invaluable in both acute and chronic myelogenous leukemias. *Symphytum* is employed more specifically for secondary cancer deposits in the bones and for tumors related to the periosteum. It has also proven of value in acute leukemia (although here it plays a secondary role to *Hekla lava*) and is particularly indicated when there has been a history of joint pain and inflammation.

> See Cases 56, 57, 59, 61, 67, 90, 91, 95, 96, 116, 118, and 121 for *Hekla lava* and 60 and 121 for *Symphytum.*

HYDRASTIS FOR CANCER OF THE STOMACH, PANCREAS, AND UPPER INTESTINAL TRACT. The remedy is also employed for cancerous affections of the mesenteric glands and the mucous membranes in general, including lungs and oesophagus. The characteristics of this remedy include yellow, thick, ropy secretions, distended abdomen, profuse perspiration, extreme weakness, and intense pain.

> See Cases 31, 33, 34, 78, 93, and 106.

LACHESIS AND *LILIUM TIGRINUM* FOR CANCER OF THE UTERUS, OVARY, AND CERVIX. Both remedies are invaluable, but *Lachesis* is more often left-sided and *Lilium tigrinum* right-sided. In the mental sphere, *Lachesis* is more loquacious, aggressive, demanding—with a heightened imagination; *Lilium tigrinum* is more prone to small anxieties, weepy—and with a "bearing down" sensation of the abdominal organs.

> See Cases 52 and 87 for *Lachesis* and Cases 49 and 55 for *Lilium tigrinum.*

Lachesis has also a strong affinity with the throat area.

> See Cases 17, 19, and 71.

LYCOPODIUM FOR LUNG CANCER. This remedy is often called for both primary and secondary deposits in the lungs. The symptoms tend to be right-sided—and frequently there is a late afternoon or early evening aggravation (4 to 8 p.m.).

See Cases 27, 28, 29, 30, 74, and 75.

The remedy is also effective in cancers of the liver, colon and prostate.

See Cases 8, 40, 46, and 84.

NITRICUM ACIDUM FOR CANCER OF THE RECTUM. Other specific areas of cancerous affections benefitted by this remedy are the mucocutaneous junctions, such as the mouth, lips, anal margin, urethra, vagina, and vulval margins. Symptoms are ulcerous eruptions and needle-like pricking pains.

See Cases 42 and 43.

ORNITHOGALUM UMBELLATUM Ø* FOR SYMPTOMATIC RELIEF IN STOMACH CANCER. Symptoms are constant pain in the stomach which is worse with eating; distention; belching of offensive flatus; vomiting of coffee-ground-like matter. The tincture can be taken in conjunction with other stomach cancer remedies as follows: 6 drops in ½ oz. of water, three or four times a day, shortly after meals.

See Cases 32 and 105.

PHOSPHORUS, although not strictly speaking an organ-specific remedy, possesses a highly specific role in the treatment of HEMORRHAGING OF CANCEROUS TUMORS OR ULCERS. Like *Sanguinaria,* it is a prime remedy to arrest internal or external bleeding *(see Chapter 7).*

See Cases 14 and 93.

Phosphorus is also employed fairly frequently in cancers of the throat area and occasionally in cancers of the female organs.

See Cases 72, 97, and 100 for throat area and Cases 4 and 120 for female organs.

---

*The symbol ø stands for the mother tincture of the remedy.

PHYTOLACCA FOR CANCERS OF THE BREAST AND PAROTID GLAND. The breast can be hard, painful, and of purple hue in later stages, with enlarged axillary glands. Often there is swelling and induration of affected glands.

> See Case 20 for parotid gland and Case 104 for the breast.

PLUMBUM IODATUM FOR CANCERS OF THE BRAIN. This remedy is of great value in tumors and cancerous growths arising out of nerve cells, especially those of the brain. *Plumbum iodatum* is preferred over *Plumbum metallicum,* because the iodide component is of particular assistance in neoplasms and any consequent infections—although, because of their close similarity, the latter can be substituted when the former is unavailable and can be, at times, preferable. For the role of *Plumbum iodatum* in Stage IV cancers, see Chapter 6.

> See Cases 11, 12, and 108.

PULSATILLA NIGRICANS AND *SEPIA* FOR CANCERS OF THE BREAST, UTERUS, OVARY, AND CERVIX. Since these remedies are usually prescribed on the basis of their "constitutional" picture as well as for their specificity for the female reproductive organs, in the following pages their well-known characteristics will be described in the individual cases benefitted by these remedies.

> See Cases 25, 53, 94, and 104 for *Pulsatilla;* and Cases 26, 50, 54, and 98 for *Sepia.*

SABAL SERRULATA FOR CANCER OF THE PROSTATE. Symptoms are prostate enlargement and a loss of sexual desire; also a history of promiscuity and/or venereal infections.

> See Cases 48 and 124.

SANGUINARIA, like *Phosphorus,* although not exactly an organ-specific remedy, IS A HIGHLY EFFECTIVE MEDICINE FOR CONTROL OF BLEEDING OF CANCEROUS TUMORS AND ULCERS. Apart from its important role in acute conditions of hemorrhage, the remedy displays symptoms of hot flushing and burning pains. It is most often used in breast and bronchogenic carcinomas.

See Cases 30, 75, and 103.

TEREBINTHINA FOR CANCER OF THE BLADDER. Symptoms are bleeding and burning pains; and difficult, scant, or painful urination.

See Cases 44, 101, and 112.

In the pages that follow, apart from *Carcinosin* and *Scirrhinum,* the reasoning behind the selection of the most appropriate (most "similar") remedy can be only cursorily indicated. For confirmation of his or her prescribing, the practitioner is urged to consult basic homoeopathic texts such as William Boericke's *Materia Medica and Repertory* and James Tyler Kent's *General Repertory of the Homoeopathic Materia Medica* (see Bibliography of Works Cited).

Method of Administration

The remedies discussed in this chapter are best prescribed in the following manner:

✦ The first prescription should be a medicine known to possess an affinity with the primary organ or to the organ at present affected—in other words, an organ-specific remedy or one of the wide-spectrum cancer specifics.

✦ The second prescription should be the appropriate cancer nosode, which is prescribed alternately (usually on alternate weeks) with the organ-specific remedy.

✦ Thereafter, and for as long as there is improvement, these two remedies are continued in weekly alternation.

N.B. In the cases that follow, the italicized information was elicited from Western tests and procedures and allopathic observation, apart from the homoeopathic interviews and treatment.

CASE 1   *September, 1995*

Male, 52 years, presented with a recurrence of a cancer of the prostate, Stage III. The tumor was 6 cm., and there were four abnormal lymph nodes in the presacral region approximately ½ cm. in size.

> *History: Earlier in 1994, the patient had undergone a transurethral resection of the prostate (TURP), followed by radiation therapy.*

PRESCRIPTION

Week 1:   *Conium* 200c - daily, Plussing Method

Week 2:   *Scirrhinum* 200c - daily, Plussing Method

Weeks 3-12:   Same as Weeks 1-2*

> *December, 1995: CT scan showed no trace of abnormal lymph nodes.*

Months 4-10:   Same as Weeks 1-2

> *Examination and tests showed no trace of tumor.*

The doctor felt secure that the case had stabilized and thereafter, the patient received *Conium* 1M and *Scirrhinum* 1M, alternating monthly, Split Dose Method. By mid-1998, treatment was stopped and there has been no trace of recurrence to date.

REMARKS

In prostate cancer, *Scirrhinum* is prescribed more often than *Carcinosin* because usually the tumors are hard.

---

*The expression "Same as" indicates that a specific procedure is to be followed for the entire period (either weeks or months)—*not* just for the first two weeks.

✦ At times (although very infrequently in recent years), the alternation of remedies need not be on a weekly basis.

CASE 2   *April, 1990*

Female, 32 years, presented with a 2 cm. lump in the left breast, in the upper left quadrant. It was freely mobile and no axillary glands were felt.

> *CT scan showed surrounding organs clear, but biopsy revealed adenocarcinoma of the breast, Stage I. Patient refused to have a lumpectomy.*

The patient had a strong family history of cancer.

PRESCRIPTION

Weeks 1-4:	*Conium* 200c - once a week, Split Dose Method
Week 5:	*Carcinosin* 200c - once, Split Dose Method Lump felt smaller.
Weeks 6-10:	Same as Weeks 1-5, alternating four weekly doses of *Conium* with one dose of *Carcinosin* Lump was 50% reduced.
Weeks 11-25:	Same as Weeks 1-5

By the end of September, 1990, the lump was fully gone and, for the next year, the patient received alternating monthly doses of *Conium* 1M and *Carcinosin* 1M, Split Dose Method. After eighteen months, all treatment stopped, and the patient is doing well to date.

REMARKS

Carcinosin was selected over *Scirrhinum* because of the family history of cancer (see p. 6).

✦ Once the cancer is stabilized or to all appearances has healed, then the two remedies can be prescribed less frequently—alternating on a semimonthly, monthly (as seen in Cases 1 and 2), two monthly, or three monthly basis—usually Split Dose Method.

CASE 3   *January, 1997*

Female, 46 years, presented with a cancer of the cervix. Three years previously she had been operated on for cancer of the rectum. No discernible metastasis at that time and patient did well during those three years.

> *A routine gynecological examination showed an ulceration on the cervix. Pathology report: squamous cell carcinoma, Stage IIa.*

PRESCRIPTION

Week 1:   *Aurum muriaticum natronatum* 200c - daily, Plussing Method

Week 2:   *Scirrhinum* 200c - daily, Plussing Method

Weeks 3-8:   Same as Weeks 1-2
               Patient felt better.

> *Examination showed ulcer to be marginally better.*

Months 3-4:   Same as Weeks 1-2

> *Examination showed ulcer continuing to improve.*

Months 5-6:   Same as Weeks 1-2

> *Examination showed ulcer to be almost 100% healed.*

Months 7-9:   Same as Weeks 1-2

> *Examination showed ulcer to be entirely healed.*

Thereafter, the woman continued visits to the doctor at three-month intervals, and alternately received a dose of *Aurum muriaticum natronatum* 200c or *Scirrhinum* 200c, Split Dose Method.

She continues to do well on the same regimen to this day.

REMARKS

In this case, *Scirrhinum* was chosen over *Carcinosin* because of her previous cancer of the rectum. Dr. Ramakrishnan has found the former to be more beneficial for rectal cancer.

For the choice of *Aurum muriaticum natronatum,* see Chapter 2.

Because, in homoeopathic prescribing, experience plays a large role in the selection of potencies, the questions of what potency to use or when to move up or down the scale of dilutions have never been easy ones.* But for the most part in treating cancer, the 200th centesimal (or 200C) is consistently Dr. Ramakrishnan's preferred potency. *Certainly, this is the dilution with which to start.* Then, over the course of months or years and as the patient improves, the prescriber moves up to the 1M, then 10M, dilution. (For a more detailed discussion of this subject, see "The Potencies" section in Chapter 7.)

---

*The homoeopathic remedies are prepared according to a specific method of diluting substances. Tinctures are diluted with alcohol and solid substances are crushed to a powder and diluted with milk sugar on a ratio of 1:10 (the x potencies) or 1:100 (the c potencies); then the process is repeated three, six, twelve, thirty, two hundred (or more) times. This method was originally introduced by Hahnemann to diminish aggravations. With each successive dilution, the liquids are succussed (strongly shaken) and the solids are triturated (ground even finer) so as to further release the "energy" of the medicine. During the process of diluting the medicinal substances, Hahnemann discovered that, paradoxically, dilution actually *increases* their curative powers. Hence the medicinal preparations are called "potencies," and the higher potencies are both the more diluted substances *and* the stronger acting ones.

Chapter 3
General Rules for the Application of the Ramakrishnan Method

The Ramakrishnan Method varies somewhat according to the stage and nature of the disease but, speaking in general terms, it can be broken down into the following procedures:

✦ In the earlier stages of the cancer (Stage I or II), if the tumor has been excised or is still small, not fixed, and no lymph glands or surrounding areas are affected (or only one or two abnormal lymph nodes are discerned), then, as was indicated in the previous chapter, the treatment begins with an organ-specific remedy and a cancer nosode, alternating the two on a weekly basis, using the daily Plussing Method. The condition is reevaluated every few weeks. Within two to four months, one should witness a reduction in the size of the tumor and/or tests showing improvement (or continuing normal), as well as improvement in the patient's sense of well-being. This procedure is continued (raising the potency if necessary) for as long as there is improvement or until the desired results are achieved.

✦ Once the critical stage is overcome and the disease has been controlled with surgery or homoeopathy or a combination of the two (i.e., the tumor is eradicated or diminished and the condition stabilized) the two remedies are administered less frequently—on a weekly, semimonthly, or monthly basis—employing the Split Dose Method. Or, if the prescriber is trained in classical constitutional prescribing, then he might choose to administer a constitutional remedy in alternation with one of the cancer remedies.

Because one never knows for certain if the cancer has been entirely eradicated or whether it might recur, follow-through is at least six months. Normally, one continues for a year or two—or even longer. The two cases that follow provide clear examples of these procedures.

CASE 4   *April, 1995*

Female, 35 years, presented with a large, hard lump (5 cm. in diameter) in her left breast. Otherwise she was physically healthy.

> *Biopsy report: adenocarcinoma, Stage II. Surgery was strongly advised, but the patient refused even a simple lumpectomy. She agreed to a CT scan, where all organs, bones, and surrounding areas showed clear.*

The woman was tall and thin, with large, lustrous eyes, obviously bright, and of an impressionable disposition—and she admitted to an overriding fear of losing the love of her boyfriend of five years; all symptoms pointing to *Phosphorus*.

PRESCRIPTION

Week 1:   *Phosphorus* 200c† (see *N.B.* on p. 21) – daily, Plussing Method

Week 2:   *Scirrhinum* 200c – daily, Plussing Method

Weeks 3-4:   Same as Weeks 1-2
             At the end of four weeks, the lump had decreased in size and was softer.

Month 2:   Same as Weeks 1-2
             Lump was 75% smaller.

Month 3:   Same as Weeks 1-2
             Lump had disappeared.

             CT scan clear and all test results normal.

Months 4-6: Same as Weeks 1-2

For two years after this, the patient received *Phosphorus* 200c and *Scirrhinum* 200c, alternating monthly, Split Dose Method. There has been no sign of recurrence to date.

REMARKS

Phosphorus was prescribed instead of an organ-specific remedy, such as *Conium* or *Phytolacca,* not only because the woman's constitutional picture stood out so clearly but also, as was mentioned in Chapter 2, because *Phosphorus* has proven to be effective in breast cancer.

In this case *Scirrhinum* was prescribed, rather than *Carcinosin,* because of the hardness of the tumor; also, Dr. Ramakrishnan often gives preference to this nosode when the patient's personality picture matches the earlier described *Phosphorus* type (see pp. 1-2; also Case 51).

N.B. *In the case examples offered throughout this book, the symbol † after a remedy indicates that it was prescribed, in part or entirely, on the basis of the "constitutional picture"—that is, on the sum total of the patient's physical, mental, and emotional symptoms, and/or personality type.*

CASE 5   *November, 1995*

Male, 54 years, a tobacco chewer, reported with an ulcer on the left margin of the tongue. The ulcer was 1 cm. in diameter, with everted margin and sloughing base, emanating a bad odor. Patient also had a swollen gland in the left cervical region and one in the submandibular region.

Biopsy report: squamous cell carcinoma, Stage II.

PRESCRIPTION

Week 1:   *Aurum muriaticum* 200c - daily, Plussing Method

Week 2:   *Carcinosin* 200C - daily, Plussing Method
                Also, *Arsenicum iodatum* 6X - twice a day.
                (Needless to say, the patient had to give up
                chewing tobacco from day one.)

Weeks 3-24:   Same as Weeks 1-2
                The ulcer was entirely healed and swelling of both
                glands had disappeared.

Months 7-9:   Same as Weeks 1-2

Months 10-18:   *Aurum muriaticum* 1M and *Carcinosin* 1M -
                alternating weekly, Split Dose Method
                Arsenicum iodatum 6X - twice a day was continued
                during the entire period

For four years, the patient has continued to receive either *Aurum muriaticum* 1M or *Carcinosin* 1M, but alternating monthly, Split Dose Method—and is perfectly healthy.

REMARKS

For the selection of *Aurum muriaticum,* see Chapter 2.

✦ For the more advanced cancer conditions (Stages III and IV)—where the primary lesion has been operated on but the excision was only partially successful, or there are widespread secondary lesions in the lymph glands or in the surrounding organs, or a cancer has recurred—the procedure is the same, but stronger measures are called for; that is, the Plussing and Split Dose Methods are employed for longer periods of time.

CASE 6   *June, 1993*

Female, 35 years, reported with a right-sided ovarian mass. She felt extremely tired and experienced severe bloating—and, since adolescence, had suffered from painful menses.

> *Patient agreed to an operation and a large (but not*
> *the entire) mass was removed, together with 30*
> *mesenteric glands, of which 13 were positive for*

malignancy. Liver and spleen were not involved. The biopsy report revealed adenocarcinoma of the ovary, Stage III. Chemotherapy and radiation therapy were advised, but the patient refused.

PRESCRIPTION

Week 1:   *Viburnum prunifolium* 200c - daily,
                Plussing Method

Week 2:   *Carcinosin* 200c - daily, Plussing Method

Weeks 3-24:   Same as Weeks 1-2
                The patient was gradually improving in energy and feeling of well-being.

                CT scan showed clear.

Months 7-12:   Same as Weeks 1-2, but in the 1M potency
                The patient continued to improve.

                CT scan continued to show no metastasis.

Months 13-18:   Same as Months 7-12

                CT scan showed clear.

Months 19-24:   Same as Months 7-12, but alternating semimonthly, Split Dose Method

Months 25-48:   Same as Months 19-24, but alternating monthly

End of treatment, except for periodic constitutional remedies alternating with *Carcinosin*. Seven years later, the woman is still doing well—and occasional scans show everything normal.

REMARKS

Viburnum prunifolium has been found to be effective in ovarian cancer when there has been a history of severe dysmenorrhea.

(For more detailed instructions on the methods of treating a patient *immediately after* or in conjunction with Western medicine and allopathic procedures, see Chapter 8.)

✦ Certainly, good results can be obtained without use of the Plussing Method; but the prescribing is more cumbersome, as can be observed in the case example cited immediately below. Compare also the rectal cancer cases, where the Plussing Method was used in Cases 41 and 42, but not in Case 43.

CASE 7   *February, 1985*

Female, 37 years, presented with a recurring astrocytoma of the brain, Stage III. Her seizures were characterized by falling unconscious, with eyes rolling down, followed by profuse perspiration and great weakness. She also suffered from various digestive problems: lactose intolerance, nausea at the sight or smell of food, distressing pain in the stomach—all symptoms pointing to *Aethusa cynapium*.

> *History: In April, 1984, the patient was operated on for a diagnosed astrocytoma of the brain, followed by radiation treatments. There was a recurrence later in 1984—and the patient was again operated on and irradiated. When there was a second recurrence in January, 1985, the patient decided to try homoeopathy.*

The woman was mild by nature, obstinate but not self-assertive, lacking in self-esteem even though competent, and was extremely sensitive to drafts, especially after being heated—all suggestive of *Silica*.

PRESCRIPTION

Month 1:   *Aethusa cynapium* 200c - weekly, Split Dose Method
The number of seizures was reduced from eleven the previous month to six during the last month.

Month 2:   Same as Month 1
There were only two seizures this month, those lasting only a few seconds.

Month 3:   *Silica* 200c† - weekly, Split Dose Method
                 There were no more seizures.

> *CT scan showed more than 50% reduction in original size of brain lesion.*

Months 4-5:   *Aethusa cynapium* 1M - weekly, Split Dose Method

Month 6:   *Medorrhinum* 200c - weekly, Split Dose Method

> *CT scan showed that the lesion in the brain had completely disappeared.*

Months 7-18:   *Aethusa cynapium* 1M and *Medorrhinum* 1M - alternating monthly, Split Dose Method

Next 3 years: Same as Months 7-18, but alternating quarterly

Thereafter, and now for more than ten years, periodic doses of either *Aethusa, Silica,* or *Medorrhinum* (as her symptoms dictated) in the 1M potency have kept the patient healthy.

REMARKS

Aethusa cynapium is particularly effective in brain tumors when there are seizures—and especially with eyes rolling down.

In the third month, *Silica* was prescribed both because of the patient's constitutional picture and because the remedy has an affinity with seizure activity. Although the organ-specific remedy was acting well, Dr. Ramakrishnan wanted to address the patient's condition on a deeper level.

Dr. Ramakrishnan also wanted to interpose a nosode, but in 1985 he had not yet developed his method of frequently using *Carcinosin*—and *Medorrhinum* fit the case well (the patient was better by the ocean, felt better lying on her stomach, and her seizure attacks took place only during the day, never at night).

For a more detailed discussion of the use of constitutional remedies, when prescribing for cancer cases, see Chapter 7.

✦ In the most advanced or terminal stage, when the metastasis is widespread throughout the body and palliation and pain control are the principal objectives, the Plussing Method is employed for as long as it is effective. After that, the remedies are administered on an as-needed basis, as described in Chapter 6.

CASE 8   *January, 1996*

Male, 53 years, developed a sudden intolerable pain in the right upper abdominal region, with a 5:00 p.m. to 7:00 p.m. aggravation of symptoms, suggestive of *Lycopodium*. He also experienced a total loss of appetite and had lost much weight.

> *Tests showed malignant secondary deposits in the liver, Stage IV. Primary site not known.*

PRESCRIPTION

Week 1:   *Lycopodium* 200c - daily, Plussing Method

Week 2:   *Scirrhinum* 200c - daily, Plussing Method

Weeks 3-8:   Same as Weeks 1-2
               The patient was much more comfortable, with a slight return of appetite.

Months 3-4:   Same as Weeks 1-2
               The patient was now very comfortable and had gained 3 lb.

Months 5-6:   Same as Weeks 1-2
               Condition continued to be stable.

Month 7:   The patient developed a severe cough and shortness of breath, and his remedies were raised to the 1M potency. He was again comfortable.

> *CT scan indicated a deposit in right lung.*

During the next several weeks, however, the patient's condition deteriorated. He was treated with the remedies *China, Carbo vegetabilis,* and *Opium,* according to his needs *(see Chapter 6)*—and died peacefully.

REMARKS

Scirrhinum, as noted in Chapter 2, is often preferable to *Carcinosin* in liver cancer.

✦ Finally, one point of procedure should be emphasized. Dr. Ramakrishnan's Plussing Method is employed *only* in the treatment of cancer—not for other degenerative or chronic diseases. Certain *acute* conditions, such as asthma attacks, high fevers, or extreme pain (from physical injury or an ailment), might call for some variation of the plussing procedure for a short period of time. But, except in cases of cancer, the taking of "plussed" remedies on a daily basis over long periods of time can be prejudicial to a patient's health.

Chapter 4

Types of Cancer That Have Responded Well to Homoeopathy and Their Most Appropriate Remedies

The types of cancer discussed in this chapter are generally presented in the traditional order of the homoeopathic repertory, beginning from the head and proceeding down—with the more generalized conditions at the end.

Numerous types of cancer exist that are not included in this chapter; to do so would be beyond the scope of this book. In these pages are those cancers most frequently encountered in Dr. Ramakrishnan's (and in the average homeopath's) experience. The significant point here is that *the Method holds true, whatever the type.*

As the reader will gather from the documentation in italics, every patient was encouraged to find an oncologist willing to cooperate with and work in conjunction with a homeopath. Also, throughout the homoeopathic treatment, he or she was regularly and closely monitored with Western medical tests and follow-up procedures. These last, in fact, are often of great assistance to the homoeopath in his choice of remedies and decisions as to the frequency and their potency. At times, however, a patient refuses to undergo certain tests or recommended procedures, despite advice to the contrary. These instances, too, are documented. Note that unless otherwise stated, in each case cited, the patient continues to do well to date (end of Year 2000).

In the case examples presented in this book, the reader will encounter certain variations and discrepancies within the methodology. The reasons for this are as follows:

1. Dr. Ramakrishnan is constantly experimenting with and refining his prescribing procedures.

2. Some of the cases cited were treated in the days before Dr. Ramakrishnan developed and refined his Plussing Method (about 1993). They will be indicated by the symbol [p-P] to signify the pre-Plussing days. These older cases are included either for teaching purposes or to show that patients are still doing well after a decade or so.

3. For added strength, a potency may have to be changed—usually raised from the 200c to the 1M potency *(see Chapter 7).*

4. In more advanced cases, the Plussing Method might not be the most effective method of treatment and may have to be replaced with a more individual method of administering the remedies *(see Chapter 6).*

5. Since the principal tenet underlying the homoeopathic approach is *individualization,* examples of successful results in the different types of cancer with remedies not listed in this book will inevitably be encountered. The medicines suggested in these pages are those which Dr. Ramakrishnan employs most frequently and with which *he* has had best results. They are offered to the reader (and practitioner) *as a place to start— or as fallbacks* when no obvious constitutional or other organ-specific remedy is apparent.

Finally, in homoeopathy, nothing is fixed or rigidly formulated. The prescriber, ever sensitive and adapting to the individual needs of his patient, must always remain flexible in his approach. That which remains a constant in the Ramakrishnan method is acquaintance (and a familiarization) with a number of the principal remedies in the treatment of this complex disease.

N.B. In this chapter, statistical charts are offered at the end of each type of cancer. The overall number of cases treated and the "viable" ones are given in rounded numbers (the viable cases exclude those in which there was no expectation of cure). *Only the numbers of "successful" cases are precise, and the calculated "Success Rate" is based solely on viable cases.* Furthermore, in judging the numbers, several factors should be taken into consideration:

+ In the post-1993 statistics, some of the fairly recent cases are considered "successful," even though the usual span of five-year nonrecurrence (by which successful treatment is judged) has not yet elapsed.

+ Many of the patients who seek homoeopathic assistance are in the later stages of cancer—and have already exhausted traditional Western treatment procedures.

+ Poor results can be due to noncompliance: to patients not following directions, not subjecting themselves to the necessary tests, not changing their poor diet, or unhealthy lifestyle; above all, not following through with the homoeopathic treatment.

Brain

The principal remedies for brain cancer, listed in order of frequency of their use by Dr. Ramakrishnan, are *Plumbum iodatum,** *Baryta carbonica, Aethusa cynapium, Baryta iodata,* and *Zincum sulphuricum.*

CASE 9   *November, 1997*

Male child, 8 years, was brought in with a recurrence of a glioma of the parietal lobe, Stage III. He was suffering from headaches and nausea.

> *In February, 1997, a glioma was operated on, followed by six months of chemotherapy. But a recent CT scan showed a recurrence of the glioma in the same place. The boy's parents decided to try homoeopathy this time.*

The boy looked and behaved a bit backward in mental development, and his parents indicated that he had difficulty with comprehension and was a poor student.

PRESCRIPTION

Week 1:	*Baryta carbonica* 200c† - daily, Plussing Method
Week 2:	*Carcinosin* 200c - daily, Plussing Method
Weeks 3-12:	Same as Weeks 1-2

CT scan showed that the tumor had not grown.

Months 4-6:	Same as Weeks 1-2

CT scan showed that the tumor had shrunk more than 50%.

Months 7-12:	Same as Weeks 1-2, but in the 1M potency

CT scan results: almost clear.

---

*Or *Plumbum metallicum* (see p. 12).

Months 13-16: Same as months 7-12

CT scan results: completely clear.

Thereafter, and to this day, the child is on the same two remedies in the 1M potency, alternating monthly, Split Dose Method.

REMARKS

Baryta carbonica was chosen over *Aethusa cynapium, Plumbum iodatum,* or *Zincum sulphuricum,* because it fit the child's constitutional picture. With the disappearance of the headaches and the tumor, however, the child grew more alert, performed better in school, and became more articulate. Today he is completely normal.

CASE 10   *March, 1996*

Male child, 10 years, was brought in for homoeopathic treatment with a recurrence of an astrocytoma. At this time, it was not large enough for the patient to undergo surgery.

> *History: Headaches and severe vomiting that were not responding sufficiently well to homoeopathic treatment called for an MRI of the brain, which showed a lesion in the frontal lobe. This was immediately operated on and the postoperative histopathological report confirmed an astrocytoma, Stage II. Radiation therapy followed surgery, and the boy was discharged as perfectly fit. Within a month his symptoms reappeared, and the MRI showed a recurrence of the growth. The parents turned to homoeopathy.*

The boy was lactose intolerant, and whenever he drank milk he vomited almost to the point of fainting, would sometimes regurgitate his food an hour after ingesting it, and was experiencing headaches again, during which he would cry out in anguish.

PRESCRIPTION

Week 1:   *Aethusa cynapium* 200c - daily, Plussing Method

Week 2:   *Carcinosin* 200c - daily, Plussing Method

Weeks 3-8:   Same as Weeks 1-2
                The boy was totally symptom free.

                MRI showed the lesion to be definitely smaller.

Months 3-4:   Same as Weeks 1-2

                MRI showed that the lesion was completely gone.

Months 5-8:   Same as Weeks 1-2, but in the 1M potency -
                weekly, Split Dose Method
                The boy was in perfect health, attending school
                and participating in sports.

                MRI continued to show everything clear.

For another year, the young patient was kept on *Aethusa cynapium* 10M and *Carcinosin* 10M, alternating monthly, Split Dose Method. After that, he received only periodic constitutional remedies or a cancer nosode and is doing well to date.

REMARKS

Aethusa cynapium is one of the most effective remedies for brain tumors, and the boy's particular symptoms fit the picture well.

CASE 11   *November, 1996*

Male, 76 years, presented with a recurrence of a glioma that had been operated on six months earlier.

> *History: Diplopia that had come on overnight called for a head scan, which revealed a mass pressing on the right optic nerve. Surgery was performed, but the mass could not be completely removed without damaging the optic nerve. The*

*histopathological diagnosis was glioma, Stage II.
Radiation therapy followed the surgery. The patient was apparently doing well for six months, but
at the end of that time, he had a recurrence of the
diplopia, and a CT scan showed a return of the
entire mass in the same place. This is when he
turned to homoeopathy.*

The involvement of the optic nerve pointed to a brain cancer remedy with a *Plumbum* component.

PRESCRIPTION

Week 1:   *Plumbum iodatum* 200c - daily, Plussing Method

Week 2:   *Carcinosin* 200c - daily, Plussing Method

Weeks 3-8:   Same as Weeks 1-2
                The patient experienced much symptomatic
                relief.

                CT scan showed the mass to be slightly smaller.

Months 3-4:   Same as Weeks 1-2
                The patient was free of symptoms. No diplopia
                was present.

                CT scan showed that the mass had shrunk further.

Months 5-12:   Same as Weeks 1-2, but in the 1M potency

                *CT scan showed that the mass had shrunk still
                further.*

Months 13-28:   Same remedies and potency - alternating weekly,
                Split Dose Method

                The patient refused to undergo any more CT scans.

Thereafter, the patient received only occasional remedies as his
symptoms dictated, and he continues to be well to date.

CASE 12   *November, 1993*

Male, 45 years, presented with astrocytoma of the brain. The tumor was in the frontal left lobe, and the patient's movements had considerably slowed down—as had his thinking. His short-term memory was also affected.

> *History: A year and a half earlier, patient investigation revealed a space-occupying lesion, Stage II. This was operated on, diagnosed as astrocytoma, and followed by radiation therapy. Ten months later, the operation was repeated for recurrence of the tumor, followed by radiation therapy. Four months later, a CT scan picked up a second recurrence of tumor and the patient turned to homoeopathy.*

PRESCRIPTION

Week 1:   *Plumbum iodatum* 200c - daily, Plussing Method

Week 2:   *Carcinosin* 200c - daily, Plussing Method

Weeks 3-8:   Same as Weeks 1-2
                 The patient showed no improvement, so the remedy was changed.

Months 3-8:   *Baryta carbonica* 200c - daily, Plussing Method

> *Head CT scans were performed on alternate months and showed steady shrinking of the tumor.*

After eight months, there was no trace of tumor. The patient continued to be treated with semimonthly doses of *Baryta carbonica* 200c for two years, and remains well to this day.

REMARKS

In Month 3, *Baryta carbonica* was selected partly because of the patient's physical and mental symptoms, partly because of the remedy's important role in brain tumors *(see Chapter 2)*.

For additional examples of successful treatment of this type of cancer, see Cases 7 and 108.

DR. RAMAKRISHNAN'S RESULTS WITH BRAIN CANCER

	No. of Cases	No. of Viable Cases	No. of Successes	Success Rate*
Pre-Plussing (<1993)	150	30	11	37%
Plussing (≥1993)	250	100	70	70%

* See N.B. on p. 31.

Oral Cavity

The principal remedies for cancer of the oral cavity, including the tongue, listed in order of frequency of use, are *Aurum muriaticum* and *Hydrastis*.

CASE 13   *February, 1997*

Female, 52 years, who had in the past been a heavy smoker, presented with a cancerous ulcer in right cheek.

> *The results of biopsy were positive: squamous cell carcinoma, Stage II. One small submandibular gland was affected; otherwise, the ulcer was localized. Radiation therapy was recommended, but the patient refused it.*

PRESCRIPTION

Week 1:   *Aurum muriaticum* 200C - daily, Plussing Method

Week 2:   *Carcinosin* 200C - daily, Plussing Method

Weeks 3-4:   Same as Weeks 1-2
               The ulcer looked better, with signs of healing.

Months 2-4:   Same as Weeks 1-2
               The ulcer was 90% healed, and the swelling in the submandibular gland completely vanished.

Months 5-6:   Same as Weeks 1-2, but in the 1M potency
               The ulcer was totally healed.

Months 7-24:   *Aurum muriaticum* 1M and *Carcinosin* 1M - alternating monthly, Split Dose Method

For an additional year, *Aurum muriaticum* 1M and *Carcinosin* 1M were prescribed, alternating quarterly, Split Dose Method.

CASE 14 [p-P]   *March, 1992*

Male, 71 years, presented with the symptoms of difficulty swallowing, restricted movement of the tongue, and incoherent speech. Examination revealed a mass on the posterior third of the tongue, with a right-sided cervical nodule that was hard and fixed.

Tongue biopsy revealed a squamous cell carcinoma, Stage III.

The patient was often chilly, disliked drafts of air, and had been an asthmatic for many years. Attacks were accompanied by thick, viscid, greenish phlegm in his throat, which came out in long, ropy strands. He also complained of headaches localized in one small spot on the head. All symptoms pointed to *Kali bichromicum*.

PRESCRIPTION

Weeks 1-3:   *Kali bichromicum* 200C† - daily, Split Dose Method
No change.

Weeks 4-6:   *Aurum muriaticum* 200C - daily, Split Dose Method
Tongue movement was better, and speech was marginally more distinct.

Weeks 7-10:   Same as Week 4
The patient continued all-around improvement. The mass had shrunk in size; by Week 10, it was 75% cleared.

At one point, there was profuse bleeding from the mass; *Phosphorus* 200C controlled it—one dose every half-hour, ten times, to be repeated in the same manner if bleeding recurred *(see Chapter 7)*.

Weeks 11-12: Same as Week 4
The patient showed no improvement.

Months 4-6:   *Kali bichromicum* 200C - weekly, Split Dose
Method
The mass cleared 80%.

Thereafter, *Kali bichromicum* 200C, weekly, Split Dose Method, was used for eighteen months. The mass remains stable at 20% of its original size.

REMARKS

Kali bichromicum was reintroduced when the progress plateaued, because it was the closest to the patient's constitutional remedy. Earlier, the impediments were too formidable; but now, having largely cleared, he could respond to his constitutional remedy.

Today, for quicker results, Dr. Ramakrishnan would have used the remedies according to the Plussing Method, interspersed with a cancer nosode.

CASE 15   *November, 1994*

Male, 42 years, who was a tobacco chewer, presented with two cancerous ulcers on the left margin of his tongue. They were indurated and foul-smelling and had the typical everted edges and hard base. The patient also had two swollen nodes in the submandibular area.

> *The biopsy report revealed squamous cell carcinoma, Stage III. The patient opted to begin with homoeopathy.*

PRESCRIPTION

Week 1:   *Aurum muriaticum* 200C - daily, Plussing Method
The patient ceased chewing tobacco from day one.

Week 2:   *Carcinosin* 200C - daily, Plussing Method

Weeks 3-4:   Same as Weeks 1-2
                The lesion had cleared about 90%, but the sub-
                mandibular glands were only marginally smaller.

Months 2-3:   Same as Weeks 1-2
                The tongue lesion entirely cleared, but the glands
                remained 60% of their original size.

> *The glands were removed surgically and the*
> *histopathological report was negative for cancer,*
> *but the site was septic from obviously poor hygiene.*

To prevent a recurrence, the patient was kept on the same two
remedies in the 1M potency, alternating monthly, Split Dose
Method, for eighteen months.

REMARKS

Once again, the sovereign role of *Aurum muriaticum* in the treatment of cancerous affections of the oral cavity is observed.

It is also noteworthy that the homoeopathic "cancer" remedies
could not benefit the noncancerous glands as well as the cancerous ulcers on the tongue. Improved hygiene and one of the *Mercurius* medicines, like *Mercurius solubilis*, might have been the
"curatives" for these glands, had they not been removed surgically.

For additional examples of successful treatment of this type of cancer, see
Cases 5 and 106.

DR. RAMAKRISHNAN'S RESULTS WITH CANCER OF THE ORAL CAVITY

	No. of Cases	No. of Viable Cases	No. of Successes	Success Rate
Pre-Plussing (<1993)	70	45	31	69%
Plussing (≥1993)	150	95	82	86%

Larynx and Vocal Cord

The principal remedies for cancer of the larynx and vocal cords, listed in order of frequency of use, are *Thuja, Phosphorus, Argentum nitricum, Lachesis,* and *Kali bichromicum.*

CASE 16 [p-P]   *May, 1990*

Male, 70 years, a heavy smoker, presented with a hoarse voice.

> *ENT examination with indirect laryngoscopy revealed a growth on the vocal cords, and analysis of scrapings yielded a diagnosis of infiltrating squamous cell carcinoma, Stage I.*

The patient was impatient, impulsive, and suffered from claustrophobia and a fear of heights. Physically, he was heat intolerant, unsteady in his gait, and prone to tremblings when anxious or tired—all symptoms pointing to *Argentum nitricum.*

PRESCRIPTION

Week 1:	*Argentum nitricum* 200c† - once, Split Dose Method The patient quit smoking.
Week 2:	*Carcinosin* 200c - once, Split Dose Method
Weeks 3-8:	Same as Weeks 1-2 The growth was 50% resolved.
Months 3-4:	Same as Weeks 1-2 The patient experienced total relief from symptoms. *Laryngoscopy showed that the growth was completely gone.*
Months 5-8:	Same as Weeks 1-2

For one year, *Argentum nitricum* 1M and *Carcinosin* 1M were prescribed, alternating monthly, Split Dose Method.

The patient lived until 1999, when he died of a heart attack at age 79.

REMARKS

Argentum nitricum was prescribed both for the constitutional picture and because it has an affinity with various affections of the vocal cords, especially in heavy smokers. Also, performers whose vocal cords are affected from fear before a performance can be assisted by the remedy.

CASE 17   *October, 1994*

Male, 47 years, a heavy smoker, presented with a sudden hoarseness. There was no pain or discomfort, and no abnormalities of the glands could be detected on palpation.

> *ENT examination showed a flat, hard growth on a vocal cord that was still slightly mobile; biopsy of a scraping revealed squamous cell carcinoma, Stage II. No detectable secondary lesions. Radiation therapy was advised, but the patient refused it.*

The patient was loquacious, had an intolerance of tight clothes (particularly around the neck), and had a history of sleeping into an aggravation of his symptoms.

PRESCRIPTION

Week 1:   *Lachesis* 200c† - daily, Plussing Method
The patient quit smoking. There was no change in hoarseness.

Week 2:   *Lachesis* 1M - daily, Plussing Method
The hoarseness was substantially reduced.

Week 3:   *Carcinosin* 1M - daily, Plussing Method

> *ENT examination showed the lesion on the cord to be smaller, less hard, and the vocal cord more freely mobile.*

Weeks 4-8:   Same as Weeks 2-3
              The patient's voice was no longer hoarse.

              *Laryngoscopy showed that the lesion was 90%
              cleared.*

Months 3-4:   Same as Weeks 2-3

              *Laryngoscopy revealed total clearance of the vocal
              cord.*

For the next six months, a dose of *Carcinosin* 1M and *Lachesis* 1M
were prescribed, alternating semimonthly, Split Dose Method.
Thereafter, no further treatment except for occasional doses of
Lachesis 1M or *Carcinosin* 1M.

REMARKS

Lachesis was the remedy chosen because of its affinity with the
throat and vocal cords and because it fit perfectly the patient's
constitutional picture.

The change of potency in Week 2 is an instance of Dr. Ramakrishnan's experimentations with the potencies (see Case 107).

Carcinosin was chosen over *Scirrhinum,* despite the hardness of
the growth, because in Dr. Ramakrishnan's experience it is the
better nosode for all vocal cord lesions.

For an additional example of successful treatment of this type of cancer,
see Case 97.

DR. RAMAKRISHNAN'S RESULTS WITH CANCER OF THE LARYNX AND VOCAL CORD

	No. of Cases	No. of Viable Cases	No. of Successes	Success Rate
Pre-Plussing (<1993)	50	24	11	46%
Plussing (≥1993)	100	43	30	70%

Thyroid and Parotid Gland

The principal remedies for thyroid cancer, listed in order of frequency of use, are *Thuja, Spongia, Iodum,* and *Lachesis.* The organ-specific remedy for cancer of the parotid gland is often *Phytolacca.*

CASE 18   *January, 1995*

Female, 41 years, presented with a diagnosed adenocarcinoma of the left lobe of the thyroid, 0.5 cm. in diameter, Stage I. Fortunately, the tumor was close to the surface and could be monitored at each stage by palpation and visualization. Otherwise, the patient was asymptomatic.

CT scan and radioactive iodine uptake evaluation had confirmed the cancerous nature of the tumor; the treatment advocated was surgery followed by chemotherapy or radiation therapy. The patient refused all conventional treatment and turned to homoeopathy.

The woman was introverted, sensitive, uncompromising in her principles and sense of rectitude; additionally, her self-confidence was not commensurate with her abilities. Physically, every small injury had a tendency to fester, and her body had a tendency to form cysts and fatty tumors. In short, she was a typical *Silica.*

PRESCRIPTION

Week 1:   *Spongia* 200c - daily, Plussing Method

Week 2:   *Carcinosin* 200c - daily, Plussing Method

Weeks 3-16:   Same as Weeks 1-2
                The patient was monitored every month.

                The lump had shrunk by 80%.

Months 5-7:   Same as Weeks 1-2, but in the 1M potency
                The lump completely disappeared.

                CT scan of the thyroid and surrounding areas revealed no lesion.

Months 8-11:   Same as Months 5-7

Months 12-24: *Spongia* 1M and *Carcinosin* 1M - alternating monthly, Split Dose Method

> *Periodic CT scans continued to show everything clear.*

Thereafter, the patient has been on periodic doses of *Silica* 1M[†] and *Carcinosin* 1M.

REMARKS

In the beginning, *Spongia* was prescribed instead of *Silica* because it is a superior organ-specific remedy for cancers of the thyroid. Because the woman responded well to the remedy, she was kept on it until she was out of danger. After that, she was prescribed her constitutional remedy together with a cancer nosode to prevent a recurrence.

CASE 19   *September, 1995*

Female, 38 years, reported with abnormal nodular glands in the neck.

> *Radioactive iodine uptake evaluation led to suspicion that the glands were malignant. Biopsy results were positive for adenocarcinoma, Stage IIb. The hard nodule was on the left thyroid, and two abnormal lymph glands were also seen in the left cervical region.*

The pressure of the thyroid was producing changes in the patient's voice. Other symptoms were not only a natural (in this case) intolerance to tight clothes around the neck but also a long-standing intolerance of tight clothes around the waist. The patient also suffered from disturbed sleep and waking up unrefreshed; and, finally, the nodules were left-sided—all symptoms pointing to *Lachesis*.

PRESCRIPTION

Week 1:   *Lachesis* 200C† - daily, Plussing Method

Week 2:   *Scirrhinum* 200C (because of hardness of nodule)
               - daily, Plussing Method

Weeks 3-8:   Same as Weeks 1-2
               Marginal improvement was observable.

Weeks 9-16:   Same as Weeks 1-2
               There was only slight further reduction in the size
               of the glands.

Week 17:   *Conium* 200C - daily, Plussing Method

Week 18:   *Scirrhinum* 200C - daily, Plussing Method

Weeks 19-32:   Same as Weeks 17-18

               *CT scan showed a rapid reduction in the size of
               cervical nodes; the main nodule was reduced 25%.*

Months 9-12:   Same as Weeks 17-18

               *CT scan showed a slight further reduction of
               cervical nodes and the main nodule.*

Months 13-18: Same as Weeks 17-18, but in the 1M potency

               *Once again, CT scan showed a slight further re-
               duction of cervical nodes and the main nodule.*

Months 19-24: Same as Weeks 17-18, but in the 10M potency
               No observable change.

               *CT scan confirmed no further reduction in the size
               of the nodule and nodes.*

For more than five years now, the picture has remained the same:
no increase, but also no further reduction of glands. The woman
receives occasional doses of *Conium* 10M, *Scirrhinum* 10M, or
Lachesis 10M to prevent recurrence.

               *CT scan every six months shows no metastasis, and
               the condition is stable.*

REMARKS

Lachesis was originally selected in part for the patient's constitutional picture, in part because the remedy has a strong affinity with cancerous affections of the throat. But *Conium,* the wide-spectrum cancer specific, was obviously the better remedy in this case.

CASE 20   *September, 1994*

Male, 52 years, presented with a lump that had recently appeared near the right temporomandibular joint; in one month it had grown to the size of a marble. There was no pain.

> *The biopsy report was positive for cancer. No other glandular enlargement. CT scan of the head, neck, and chest showed all clear. Diagnosis: Adenocarcinoma of the parotid gland, Stage I. The patient decided to begin with homoeopathic treatment.*

The lump was hard, but not stony hard, and was freely mobile; there was no excessive salivation. The only pain the patient experienced was sometimes in the right jaw, when he had been chewing hard.

PRESCRIPTION

Week 1:	*Phytolacca* 200C - daily, Plussing Method
Week 2:	*Carcinosin* 200C - daily, Plussing Method
Weeks 3-8:	Same as Weeks 1-2 No improvement whatsoever, so some change of prescription was needed.
Months 3-4:	Same as Weeks 1-2, but in the 1M potency This time, some change was visible.
Months 5-6:	Same as Months 3-4 Further reduction in size of the tumor, but not as much as during the previous eight weeks.

Months 7-9:   Same as Weeks 1-2, but in the 10M potency
               At the end of this time, the mass had fully cleared.

Tests confirmed patient to be all clear.

Months 10-36: Same two remedies in the 10M potency, but alter-
              nating monthly, Split Dose Method

End of treatment.

REMARKS

Phytolacca, as was noted in Chapter 2, is one of the preeminent remedies for cancers of the glands, especially of the breast and parotid gland.

For an additional example of successful treatment of thyroid cancer, see Case 100.

Dr. Ramakrishnan's Results with Cancer of the Thyroid and Parotid Gland

	No. of Cases	No. of Viable Cases	No. of Successes	Success Rate
Pre-Plussing (<1993)	25	12	7	58%
Plussing (≥1993)	40	17	12	71%

Oesophagus

The principal remedies for cancer of the oesophagus, listed in order of frequency of use, are *Causticum, Thuja, Argentum nitricum, Silica,* and *Arsenicum album.*

CASE 21 [p-P]   *May, 1990*

Male, 45 years, presented with an inability to swallow that had been gradually increasing over a two-month period.

> *Endoscopy revealed an ulceration in the oesopha-gus; biopsy reported squamous cell carcinoma, Stage II, with surrounding organs and area all clear.*

The patient was of a sociable disposition, ever ready to help out those in need. Physically, he had warts on the face and fingers, and a slight facial palsy.

PRESCRIPTION

Weeks 1-4:   *Causticum* 200c† - Split Dose Method, once a week

Week 5:   *Carcinosin* 200c - Split Dose Method, once

Weeks 6-14:   Same as Weeks 1-5
By the end of three and a half months, the patient could eat normally.

Months 3-6:   Same as Weeks 1-5

> *Endoscopy showed the ulcer completely healed.*

Months 7-9:   Same as Weeks 1-5

For one more year, single doses of *Causticum* 1m and *Carcinosin* 1m were prescribed, alternating monthly, Split Dose Method.

REMARKS

Causticum was prescribed because the remedy fit the patient's constitutional picture, and because, although it is not, strictly speaking, an organ-specific remedy, it has a definite affinity with the throat, larynx, and oesophagus.

CASE 22 [p-P]   *November, 1991*

Male, 60 years, reported with a gradually worsening dysphagia, so that now he could only swallow liquids and finely mashed rice.

> *An endoscope could not pass beyond the mid-third of the oesophagus; biopsy showed squamous cell carcinoma, Stage III. CT scan indicated that the liver, pancreas, and spleen were not affected, but x-ray evaluation of the chest showed secondary lesions in the lungs and the seventh right rib.*

The patient was sensitive, soft spoken, and conscientious from childhood; he would make great efforts to work hard but lacked stamina. He was never a good eater and always had a poor digestion. He was chilly but liked cold food and drink and was lactose intolerant.

PRESCRIPTION

Weeks 1-2:	*Silica* 200c† - Split Dose Method, once a week
Week 3:	*Conium* 200c - Split Dose Method, once
Weeks 4-6:	Same as Weeks 1-3 Only slight improvement was reported.
Weeks 7-9:	Same as Weeks 1-3, but with *Silica* in the 1M potency Marginal improvement continued.
Weeks 10-12:	Same as Weeks 7-9 By this time, the patient was able to eat almost normally but still needed soft foods. Improvement was noticeable but slow.
Weeks 13-21:	Same as Weeks 1-3, but with *Silica* in the 10M potency (to speed up improvement)

Week 22:   The patient developed obstructive symptoms that looked like a recurrence. But Dr. Ramakrishnan, suspecting a stricture due to fibrosis from the clearing of the oesophageal neoplasms, gave him a Split Dose of *Causticum* 200c (see pp. 198-200).

> *During Week 23, endoscopy confirmed that the man was 90% cleared and only fibrosis was present; it was cleared by the endoscope.*

Weeks 24-52:   Same as Weeks 13-21

For two more years, the patient received periodic doses of *Silica* 10M. Then all treatment stopped when the patient moved. He still calls in to report that he remains healthy.

REMARKS

Silica was prescribed not only for the patient's constitutional picture, but also because the remedy has an affinity with the periosteum and bones.

Conium, as noted in Chapter 2, is an excellent remedy for secondary lesions in the bones.

Today, Dr. Ramakrishnan would have also employed a cancer nosode.

DR. RAMAKRISHNAN'S RESULTS WITH CANCER OF THE OESOPHAGUS

	No. of Cases	No. of Viable Cases	No. of Successes	Success Rate
Pre-Plussing (<1993)	90	58	31	53%
Plussing (≥1993)	210	110	88	80%

Mediastinum

The principal remedies for mediastinal cancer, listed in order of frequency of use, are *Thuja, Spongia,* and *Scrophularia nodosa.*

CASE 23   *October, 1998*

Female, 63 years, sought homoeopathic treatment for a cancerous supraclavicular gland.

> *A stony-hard gland had been surgically removed earlier that year; the biopsy report revealed a squamous cell carcinoma, Stage III. The primary tumor was not detectable. The gland returned and the patient then turned to homoeopathy.*

The patient had a history of asthma, numerous warts, and periodic fibroadenosis of the breast.

PRESCRIPTION

Week 1:   *Thuja* 200c† - daily, Plussing Method

Week 2:   *Scirrhinum* 200c - daily, Plussing Method

Weeks 3-12:   Same as Weeks 1-2

> *CT scan showed considerable regression of the gland.*

Months 4-6:   Same as Weeks 1-2, but in the 1M potency.

> *CT scan showed that the supraclavicular area had completely cleared.*

Month 7:   *Thuja* 1M - semimonthly, Split Dose Method

Month 8:   *Scirrhinum* 1M - semimonthly, Split Dose Method

Months 9-18:   Same as Months 7-8.
              The intensive treatment ended. Now the patient receives only periodic doses of *Thuja* 1M or *Scirrhinum* 1M.

REMARKS

Thuja was prescribed partly on the basis of the woman's symptomatic picture (past and present) and partly on the basis of the remedy's affinity for affections of the glands in general.

Scirrhinum was the nosode selected because of the stony hardness of the original gland.

CASE 24   *September, 1995*

Male, 52 years, came to homoeopathy for adenocarcinoma of glands in the mediastinum—with an enlargement of the neck, a bulging left carotid artery, and some varicosity in the veins of the neck. His present symptoms were a continuous cough with little expectoration, which was worse when he was lying down; he had shortness of breath, even when at rest, which was worse after coughing, talking, drinking hot liquids, and from worry.

> *CT scan of lungs, echocardiography, and other tests disclosed multiple enlarged glands in the mediastinum. Biopsy of a piece of removed gland revealed adenocarcinoma, Stage III. Radiation therapy was advised, but the patient refused.*

PRESCRIPTION

Weeks 1-2:   *Spongia* 30c - for relief of cough
To be taken at first more frequently, several times a day, then on an as-needed basis. Cough was much relieved.

Week 3:   *Carcinosin* 200c - daily, Plussing Method

Week 4:   *Spongia* 200c - daily, Plussing Method

Weeks 5-6:   Same as Weeks 3-4
Cough 90% better; only occasional dyspnea.

Weeks 7-10:   Same as Weeks 3-4

> *CT scan showed glands reduced about 25% of original size.*

Weeks 11-18:   Same as Weeks 3-4

> *CT scan indicated that the glands remained the same size; a scan of the liver, spleen, and pancreas and blood workups showed everything clear.*

In January, 1996, the patient stopped coming for homoeopathic treatment. But in December, 1997, after having vanished for almost two years, he returned when his cough reappeared.

> *CT scan showed the glands to be just the same— neither grown nor shrunk; all other indicators appeared normal.*

PRESCRIPTION

Week 1:   *Spongia* 200c - daily, Plussing Method

Week 2:   *Carcinosin* 200c - daily, Plussing Method

Weeks 3-8:   Same as Weeks 1-2
The patient reported that he was feeling very hot and was craving air conditioning (which he never previously needed) and the blast of a fan.

Week 9:   *Iodum* 200c - daily, Plussing Method

Week 10:   *Carcinosin* 200c - daily, Plussing Method

Weeks 11-12:   Same as Weeks 9-10
The patient reported feeling much better ("as if a big load is off my chest"). Neck swelling was almost gone.

Month 4:   Same as Weeks 9-10
The patient continued to feel better.

> *CT scan showed no change.*

Months 5-10:   Same as Weeks 9-10

> *CT scan showed the size and number of glands significantly reduced. Of eight nodes seen originally, only three remained—and these were only half the original size.*

At this point, the patient got tired of the Plussing Method and refused to continue it. Thus, for the next year, he was put on *Iodum* 1M and *Carcinosin* 1M—alternating weekly, Split Dose Method. The following year, remedies prescribed were the same, but in the 10M potency.

REMARKS

This case exemplifies the necessity of carrying through with a case, even when there is marked improvement. Otherwise, there is danger of a recurrence.

Iodum was prescribed because of the patient's unusual temperature modality (extremely hot) and because it is a prime remedy for glands.

Spongia was initially prescribed for its affinity with the patient's symptoms as well as with the mediastinal area.

For an additional example of successful treatment of "secondary adenitis," or cancerous glands in the general mediastinal area, see Case 113.

Dr. Ramakrishnan's Results with Mediastinal Cancer

	No. of Cases	No. of Viable Cases	No. of Successes	Success Rate
Pre-Plussing (<1993)	20	9	3	33%
Plussing (≥1993)	40	22	16	73%

Breast

The principal remedies for breast cancer, listed in order of frequency of use, are *Conium, Pulsatilla, Sepia, Phytolacca,* and *Phosphorus.*

CASE 25   *January, 1995*

Female, 39 years, presented with a 1 cm. lump in the right breast, lower quadrant, that had been diagnosed as cancerous, Stage II. One abnormal axillary lymph node was found; no other sign of metastasis. The woman refused a lumpectomy and turned to homoeopathy instead.

> *History: To regulate painful and irregular menstrual periods, the patient had undergone hormonal treatment several times.*

The patient was overweight, could eat only a little at a time, but liked pastries; she was easily chilled but craved fresh air. She was gentle by nature; easily felt hurt or slighted; and was low-spirited, mornings and evenings—all symptoms pointing to *Pulsatilla.*

PRESCRIPTION

Week 1:   *Pulsatilla* 200C† - daily, Plussing Method

Week 2:   *Carcinosin* 200C - daily, Plussing Method

Weeks 3-8:   Same as Weeks 1-2
               Slight reduction in the size of the lump.

> *CT scan confirmed that the tumor was reduced by 25%.*

Months 3-6:   Same as Weeks 1-2, but in the 1M potency
               By the end of this time, the lump had disappeared and the lymph node appeared normal.

> *CT scan showed everything clear.*

Months 7-10:   Same as Weeks 1-2, but in the 10M potency—weekly, Split Dose Method

Thereafter, and for the next two years, the woman was prescribed alternating monthly doses of *Pulsatilla* 10M and *Carcinosin* 10M, Split Dose Method. During this time her menstrual periods became regular and pain free.

REMARKS

In this case, *Pulsatilla* served both as an organ-specific and constitutional remedy.

CASE 26   *March, 1996*

Female, 41 years, presented with a 2 cm. lump in the right breast, lower quadrant, which had been diagnosed as cancerous, Stage II. It was freely mobile, not adherent to pectoral muscles. No axillary glands were palpable, but the patient had noticed that the lump had slowly been growing for the past six months.

CT scan revealed all surrounding organs, lungs, liver, and spleen free of tumors; bones were also clear. The patient refused to have a lumpectomy.

No clear constitutional remedy evolved from the homoeopathic consultation, but the tumor was stony hard.

PRESCRIPTION

Week 1:	*Conium* 200C - daily, Plussing Method
Week 2:	*Scirrhinum* 200C - daily, Plussing Method
Weeks 3-12:	Same as Weeks 1-2
	CT scan revealed a 50% decrease in size of tumor.
Months 4-6:	Same as Weeks 1-2
	CT showed no further reduction.
Months 7-10:	Same as Weeks 1-2, but in the 1M potency
	CT still showed no further reduction.

For one more year, the same two remedies in the 1M potency, alternating monthly, Split Dose Method, were prescribed. Thereafter, and to this day, the patient receives quarterly doses of *Sepia* 200c†, Split Dose Method.

After four years, no metastasis was found anywhere, the axillary glands were clear, but the primary lump remains about 50% of its original 2 cm. size.

> *For one year, a CT scan was repeated every three months to watch for signs of metastasis. After that, scanning was performed only occasionally.*

REMARKS

Sepia was prescribed because of the patient's food preferences and liking for vigorous exercise; also her reserved, self-contained, but forthright nature (all of which manifested over time) pointed to this remedy.

For additional examples of successful treatment of this type of cancer, see Cases 2, 4, 94, and 98.

Dr. Ramakrishnan's Results with Breast Cancer

	No. of Cases	No. of Viable Cases	No. of Successes	Success Rate
Pre-Plussing (<1993)	190	70	40	57%
Plussing (≥1993)	380	150	120	80%

Lung

The principal remedies for lung cancer, listed in order of frequency of use, are *Lycopodium, Kali bichromicum, Argentum nitricum,* and *Lachesis.*

CASE 27   *November, 1995*

Male, 51 years, presented with an incessant cough, which he had had for the past month. He had been a smoker for twenty years but had stopped ten years previously.

> *Bronchoscopy revealed a lesion in the right upper lobe and four abnormal paratracheal lymph nodes; a subsequent workup revealed squamous cell carcinoma, Stage III.*

The patient was lean, flatulent, with a history of early graying of his hair. He liked privacy but disliked being alone in the house. He was intellectual, with a mind of his own, but respectful of those in authority.

PRESCRIPTION

Week 1:   *Lycopodium* 200c† - daily, Plussing Method

Week 2:   *Scirrhinum* 200c - daily, Plussing Method

Weeks 3-4:   Same as Weeks 1-2
               Cough was considerably reduced.

Weeks 5-8:   Same as Weeks 1-2

> *CT scan showed that the lesion and paratracheal nodes had shrunk 10%.*

Weeks 9-10:   Same as Weeks 1-2, but in the 1M potency

Weeks 11-16:   Same as Weeks 9-10

> *CT scan showed the lesion and nodes had shrunk to 25% of their original size.*

Months 5-6:   Same as Weeks 9-10
                The patient was completely asymptomatic.

                *CT scan showed the lesion and nodes had shrunk
                to 10% of their original size.*

Months 7-12:   Same as Weeks 9-10

Month 13:   *Lycopodium* 1M - semimonthly, Split Dose
                Method

Month 14:   *Scirrhinum* 1M - semimonthly, Split Dose Method

Months 15-24:   Same as Months 13-14

For two more years, the patient was given alternate monthly doses of the two remedies, Split Dose Method. He did not want to undergo any more CT scans after the six-month evaluation but is reporting regularly to the doctor and is doing well.

REMARKS

Lycopodium, as noted in Chapter 2, can be considered an organ-specific remedy for lung cancer. The remedy also perfectly fit the patient's personality and constitutional type.

CASE 28   *September, 1994*

Male, 61 years, presented with a history of thyroid cancer that had metastasized to the right upper lobe of the lung.

> *History: A hard lump on the right side of thyroid gland had within six months grown to the size of a lemon. It was diagnosed as adenocarcinoma of the thyroid gland, Stage IIIa. The tumor was excised surgically, followed by radiation therapy. The patch on the upper lobe of the lung remained static despite all treatment.*

PRESCRIPTION

Week 1:	*Lycopodium* 200C - daily, Plussing Method
Week 2:	*Carcinosin* 200C - daily, Plussing Method
Weeks 3-16:	Same as Weeks 1-2

> *Tests showed the lesion in the lung had cleared almost 90%.*

Months 5-8:	Same as Weeks 1-2, but in the 1M potency.

> *Tests showed the lesion in the lung completely cleared.*

Since Month 8, and to this day, the patient has been kept on *Lycopodium* 1M and *Carcinosin* 1M, alternating monthly, Split Dose Method.

REMARKS

Despite the hardness of the original lump, *Carcinosin* was chosen rather than *Scirrhinum*, because the original site of the cancer was in the thyroid gland, for which condition *Carcinosin* has proven to be the more suitable nosode.

CASE 29   *July, 1995*

Male, 85 years, presented with shortness of breath, a cough with hard, tenacious (ropy), bloodstained expectoration, and loss of weight. This had been going on for six months and had been especially acute during the past three months.

> *Tests confirmed a bronchogenic carcinoma in the left lower lobe of the lung, Stage III. The aspirated epithelial fluid was denoting either a primary or secondary lesion. The patient refused all treatment except homoeopathy.*

PRESCRIPTION

Week 1: *Kali bichromicum* 200c - daily, Plussing Method

Week 2: *Carcinosin* 200c - daily, Plussing Method

Weeks 3-4: Same as Weeks 1-2
Bleeding completely stopped.

Weeks 5-22: Same as Weeks 1-2
The patient felt much better.

> *X-ray evaluations in December, 1995, and
> January, 1996, showed steady improvement.*

At one point during this time, the patient became very depressed, irritable, and uncommunicative; his mood worsened in the late afternoons and early evenings. *Lycopodium* 200c, one dose every hour for ten hours, pulled him out of his low mood.

Months 6-16: Same as Weeks 1-2, but in the 1M potency

> *X-ray evaluation showed the lung almost clear.*

Months 17-26: Same as Weeks 1-2, but in the 10M potency

> *X-ray evaluation showed the lung entirely clear.*

For eighteen months the patient received *Kali bichromicum* 10M and *Carcinosin* 10M, alternating semimonthly, Split Dose Method. Then intensive treatment ended, and today he receives only an occasional dose of either remedy.

REMARKS

Kali bichromicum was prescribed in part for the patient's type of expectoration, in part because of the remedy's important role in the treatment of lung cancer.

CASE 30   *November, 1995*

Male, 68 years, a heavy smoker for most of his life, presented with an incessant cough and unbearable pain in the interscapular region.

> *X-ray evaluation showed consolidation in the right lower lobe of the lungs; a scan confirmed this and a bronchoscopy with brushings of the bronchi revealed the presence of malignant cells. Diagnosis: bronchogenic carcinoma, Stage III.*

The patient was haughty and reserved by nature, craved sweets, and was in other respects a typical *Lycopodium* (see Case 27).

PRESCRIPTION

Week 1:   *Lycopodium* 200c† - daily, Plussing Method

Week 2:   *Carcinosin* 200c - daily, Plussing Method

Weeks 3-8:   Same as Weeks 1-2

Months 3-4:   Same as Weeks 1-2, but in the 1M potency
                 Twice during these weeks, the patient developed hemoptysis and both times *Sanguinaria* 200c—a dose every half-hour, ten times, which he repeated for three successive days—pulled him through (see p. 183).

> *CT scan showed the entire patch of consolidation completely cleared.*

Months 5-6:   Same as Weeks 1-2

Months 7-12:   Same as Weeks 1-2, but in the 1M potency

> *CT scan continued to show everything clear.*

Month 13:   *Lycopodium* 1M, semimonthly, Split Dose Method

Month 14:   *Carcinosin* 1M, semimonthly, Split Dose Method

Months 15-26:   Same as Months 13-14

> *All this time the patient was symptom free (no*
> *blood in sputum, etc.), but he refused to undergo*
> *any more bronchoscopies or other tests.*

For one more year, the patient received the same two remedies, alternating quarterly, Split Dose Method, and thereafter, only occasionally. He continues well to this day, with no cough or other symptoms.

> *Recent CT scan shows everything clear.*

REMARKS

In this case, *Carcinosin* was prescribed, rather than *Scirrhinum* (as in Case 27), because there was a family history of cancer, which *(as mentioned in Chapter 2)* is a strong indication for *Carcinosin*.

It is noteworthy how strongly *Lycopodium* predominates when the lung cancer is right-sided.

For an additional example of successful treatment of this type of cancer, see Case 107.

Dr. Ramakrishnan's Results with Lung Cancer

	No. of Cases	No. of Viable Cases	No. of Successes	Success Rate
Pre-Plussing (<1993)	40	21	6	29%
Plussing (≥1993)	90	26	15	58%

Stomach

The principal remedies for stomach cancer, listed in order of frequency of use, are *Hydrastis, Cadmium sulphuratum, Arsenicum album,* and *Kali bichromicum.* Additionally, *Ornithogallum* ø, used concurrently with the remedies for pain relief, is invaluable.

CASE 31   *September, 1994*

Male, 52 years, was experiencing a burning in the stomach, which had been diagnosed as adenocarcinoma of the stomach, Stage IV.

History: Endoscopy had revealed a mass 2 inches in diameter sitting on the great curvature. Surgery had been performed to remove the entire stomach, but a CT scan revealed he had multiple cancerous mesenteric glands and secondary lesions in the spleen, liver, and lungs, which could not be removed surgically. Chemotherapy was advised, but the patient refused.

PRESCRIPTION

Week 1:	*Hydrastis* 200c - daily, Plussing Method
Week 2:	*Conium* 200c - daily, Plussing Method
Week 3:	*Carcinosin* 200c - daily, Split Dose Method The patient felt better.
Weeks 4-12:	Same as Weeks 1-3 The patient continued to feel better.
	CT scan showed no lesions (!).
Week 13:	*Hydrastis* 200c - daily, Plussing Method
Week 14:	*Carcinosin* 200c - daily, Plussing Method
Weeks 15-28:	Same as Weeks 13-14
Months 8-12:	Same as Weeks 13-14, but in the 1M potency

Months 13-15: Same as Weeks 13-14, but in the 10M potency

Three-month CT scans continued clear.

Months 16-28: *Hydrastis* 10M and *Carcinosin* 10M, alternating monthly, Split Dose Method

Six-month CT scans continued clear.

Since early 1997, the patient, who now takes the two remedies, alternating quarterly, continues to be comfortable and asymptomatic, is maintaining his weight, and attends to two to three hours of business every day.

REMARKS

This is a rare instance in which Dr. Ramakrishnan started out with three remedies.

Hydrastis was chosen because it is a major remedy for stomach cancer and other abdominal organs.

Conium was chosen because of its affinity for cancers of the glands, particularly when they are very hard, as they were in this case; also because the remedy is good for cancers of the stomach and abdominal organs. But since, according to the patient, *Conium* offered less symptomatic relief than the other two remedies, it was dropped after the twelfth week.

Carcinosin was chosen rather than *Scirrhinum,* because it is the preferred nosode in cancers of the abdominal organs, except for the liver.

CASE 32   *February, 1994*

Male, 77 years, reported to homoeopathy with loss of appetite and of weight, disturbed sleep, and much weakness from a stomach cancer.

> *Endoscopic findings were a nodular mass involving the antrum of the stomach, Stage III. The scope could not pass beyond the duodenum.*

The patient was highly sensitive to the cold, fastidious in all matters, was definitely a "morning" person, and had a critical and commanding personality—a typical *Arsenicum album* type.

PRESCRIPTION

Week 1:   *Arsenicum album* 200c† - daily, Plussing Method

Week 2:   *Carcinosin* 200c - daily, Plussing Method
               Also, *Ornithogalum* ø, for pain or discomfort, several times a day.

Weeks 3-24:   Same as Weeks 1-2
               The patient continued with *Ornithogalum* ø, as needed.

               Twice during this period, the patient received *Kali bichromicum* 200c instead of *Arsenicum album*, when the mucoid material that he threw up was greenish and stringy.

               Endoscopy showed everything normal.

Months 7-15:   Same remedies as Weeks 1-2, but in the 1M potency, alternating weekly, Split Dose Method.

Thereafter, the patient received monthly doses of either *Arsenicum album, Carcinosin,* or *Kali bichromicum,* Split Dose Method, as his symptoms dictated—and he continues well.

REMARKS

Ornithogalum ø, taken as an adjunct to the remedies, is invaluable in the treatment of cancers of the stomach *(see Chapter 2)*.

DR. RAMAKRISHNAN'S RESULTS WITH STOMACH CANCER

	No. of Cases	*No. of Viable Cases*	*No. of Successes*	*Success Rate*
Pre-Plussing (<1993)	80	23	8	35%
Plussing (≥1993)	130	55	30	55%

Pancreas

The principal remedies for pancreatic cancer, listed in order of frequency of use, are *Hydrastis, Ceanothus americanus, Arsenicum album, Cadmium sulphuratum,* and *Baryta iodata.*

CASE 33   *February, 1993*

Male, 37 years, presented with a 5 cm. cancerous mass at the head of the pancreas in the periampullary region, which had been diagnosed as Stage II.

> *Tests showed high biliary dilation, and CT scan revealed that there was total obstruction of the biliary flow. Total serum bilirubin was 7.2 mg./dL.*

PRESCRIPTION

Week 1:	*Hydrastis* 200c - daily, Plussing Method
Week 2:	*Carcinosin* 200c - daily, Plussing Method
Weeks 4-6:	Same as Weeks 1-2 The patient felt better. But on subsequent examination, the splenetic hardness was distinctive.
Week 7:	*Hydrastis* 200c - daily, Plussing Method
Week 8:	*Scirrhinum* 200c - daily, Plussing Method

> *Bilirubin count was lower.*

Months 3-4:	Same as Weeks 7-8, but in the 1M potency The patient continued to improve.

> *Bilirubin count continued to drop. CT scan showed 50% reduction in the mass, and the spleen was normal in size and texture.*

Months 5-12:	Same as Weeks 7-8 The patient felt completely well.

> *Bilirubin count was down to 1.3 mg./dL. at the end of six months and remained at that level thereafter.*

CT scan showed further marginal reduction of the pancreatic tumor.

At this point, the patient declared that he was tired of the Plussing Method and would no longer continue it. He also refused to undergo any more CT scans.

Months 13-20: Same two remedies as Weeks 7-8, but in the 10M potency - daily, Split Dose Method
The patient continued to do well.

After this, intensive treatment was discontinued and the patient now receives only periodic remedies, as his symptoms dictate.

REMARKS

Hydrastis was prescribed because it is the primary organ-specific remedy for pancreatic cancer.

Scirrhinum replaced *Carcinosin,* because the enlarged spleen was rock hard.

CASE 34   *September, 1993*

Male, 50 years, sought homoeopathic assistance for a diagnosed cancerous mass at the head of the pancreas, in the periampullary region, Stage III. The patient was jaundiced, with high biliary dilation, was vomiting blood, and was extremely weak and dejected.

Total serum bilirubin 13.2 mg./dL.; hemoglobin 4.5 gm./dL. The patient refused recommended surgery and turned to homoeopathy.

The patient displayed certain constitutional and personality characteristics suggestive of *Thuja;* an early childhood history of eczema and asthma (from vaccination?); an original, if somewhat confused and chaotic mind; and a fear of the out-of-body sensations he would occasionally experience.

PRESCRIPTION

Week 1:   *Hydrastis* 200c - daily, Plussing Method

Week 2:   *Carcinosin* 200c - daily, Plussing Method
                 The patient felt somewhat better.

Weeks 3-24:   Same as Weeks 1-2

                 *CT scan showed no evidence of pancreatic patholo-
                 gy; total serum bilirubin 2 mg./dL. and hemoglo-
                 bin 11.2 gm./dL. Scan also showed enlargement of
                 the liver, which on palpation was found to be very
                 hard.*

Weeks 25-26:   For no apparent reason the patient's condition
                 started to deteriorate; he experienced severe ab-
                 dominal pain, loss of appetite, vomiting. *Ar-
                 senicum album* 200c helped only a little. Then
                 Thuja 200c† in frequent doses was tried and the
                 patient rallied.

Week 27:   *Thuja* 200c† - daily, Plussing Method

Week 28:   *Scirrhinum* 200c - daily, Plussing Method
                 The patient continued to feel better.

Months 8-12:   Same as Weeks 27-28
                 Improvement continued.

Months 13-22:   Same as Weeks 27-28, but in the 1M potency
                 The patient was back to normal.

                 Results of blood tests and CT scan were all normal.

For two years the patient was on *Thuja* 1M and *Scirrhinum* 1M, alternating monthly, Split Dose Method. Today he is full of vigor
and enthusiasm and is enjoying life.

REMARKS

Scirrhinum was selected in Week 28 because of the hardness of the
liver.

CASE 35   *November, 1994*

Female, 60 years, came for homoeopathic treatment for her loss of appetite, nausea, and extreme weakness. She was jaundiced, had a mild fever, and claimed she had been steadily deteriorating since April, 1993. Her hemoglobin level was 6.5 gm./dL. and serum bilirubin 4.2 mg./dL.; the erythrocyte sedimentation rate (ESR) at 1 hour was 112 mm.

> *CT scan showed a nodular growth in the head of the pancreas and an enlarged liver and spleen. Laparoscopic biopsy of the head of the pancreas and histopathological evaluation confirmed squamous cell carcinoma, Stage III. The endoscope went in smoothly up to the second part of the duodenum. The ampulla looked normal, but the scope could be passed only 5 cm. and no further. Chemotherapy was advised, but the patient turned to homoeopathy instead.*

PRESCRIPTION

Week 1:   *Baryta iodata* 200c - daily, Plussing Method

Week 2:   *Carcinosin* 200c - daily, Plussing Method

                 ESR dropped from 112 mm. to 75 mm.

Weeks 3-16:   Same as Weeks 1-2

                 Tests and CT scan showed everything normal.

Months 5-12:   Same as Weeks 1-2

                 Tests and CT scan continued to show everything normal.

Months 13-30:   Same two remedies as in Weeks 1-2, but in the 1M potency, alternating monthly, Split Dose Method

Thereafter, the woman received *Baryta iodata* 1M and *Carcinosin* 1M, alternating quarterly, Split Dose Method—and continues the regimen to this day.

REMARKS

Baryta iodata was chosen because of the patient's extreme weakness, her anemia, and the remedy's affinity with the glands and endocrine organs.

For additional examples of successful treatment of this type of cancer, see Cases 102, 115, and 117.

Dr. Ramakrishnan's Results with Pancreatic Cancer

	No. of Cases	No. of Viable Cases	No. of Successes	Success Rate
Pre-Plussing (<1993)	22	10	4	40%
Plussing (≥1993)	98	56	42	75%

Liver

The principal remedies for liver cancer, listed in order of frequency of use, are *Chelidonium, Hydrastis, Lycopodium,* and *Natrum sulphuricum. Chelidonium* ø can be used concomitantly with other remedies for pain relief.

CASE 36   *March, 1995*

Female, 47 years, presented with secondary deposits in the liver (after having had breast cancer), Stage IV.

> *History: In February, 1994, results of a biopsy of a lump in the right breast were positive for cancer. A lumpectomy was performed, and seven of the sixteen axillary glands removed were positive. Both ovaries were removed, as was the uterus, which had large fibroids. Surgery was followed by chemotherapy and radiation therapy.*
>
> *In January, 1995, CT scan identified deposits on the liver. A CT scan–guided biopsy of the deposit was performed; the histopathology report was positive for malignancy. Another round of chemotherapy was advised, but the patient refused and turned to homoeopathy.*

The patient was a typical *Calcarea carbonica:* overweight, with poor muscular tone; emotional and apprehensive; conscientious in her duties, but a plodder in executing them.

PRESCRIPTION

Week 1:   *Chelidonium* 200c - daily, Plussing Method

Week 2:   *Carcinosin* 200c - daily, Plussing Method

Weeks 3-4:   Same as Weeks 1-2

> *CT scan showed deposits about the same; maybe somewhat smaller.*

Month 2:   Same as Weeks 1-2

           CT scan showed considerable reduction of deposits.

Month 3:   Same as Weeks 1-2

           CT scan showed deposits had cleared 90%.

Month 4:   *Calcarea carbonica* 200c† - weekly, Split Dose Method

Month 5:   *Carcinosin* 200c - weekly, Split Dose Method

           CT scan showed deposits cleared.

Months 6-12: Same as Months 4-5

Thereafter, the woman received *Calcarea carbonica* 200c and *Carcinosin* 200c, alternating monthly, Split Dose Method—and, to the present day, continues to do well.

           Periodic CT scans show everything is still normal.

REMARKS

This is a classic instance of how the constitutional remedy can follow an organ-specific remedy, once there is marked improvement in the organ affected *(see Chapter 7).*

Chelidonium's important role in the treatment of liver cancer is described in Chapter 2.

CASE 37   *March, 1996*

Female, 41 years, a severe diabetic, reported with a secondary cancer of the liver, which had metastasized from the left breast, Stage IV. The liver was slightly enlarged, very hard, and tender to the touch.

           History: In August, 1994, an infiltrating ductile
           carcinoma of the left breast was operated on, fol-
           lowed by chemotherapy and radiation therapy. In
           June, 1995, there was a recurrence in the same

breast. Radical mastectomy and total hysterectomy were performed, followed by chemotherapy and radiation therapy. In February, 1996, CT scan showed deposits on the liver, and a guided biopsy was positive for secondary metastatic adenocarcinoma.

PRESCRIPTION

Week 1:   *Natrum sulphuricum* 200c - daily, Plussing Method

Week 2:   *Scirrhinum* 200c - daily, Plussing Method

Weeks 3-8:   Same as Weeks 1-2
                Tenderness of the liver was completely gone.

                CT scan showed the deposits smaller, the liver normal size.

Months 3-4:   Same as Weeks 1-2

                CT scan showed that the liver secondaries had completely disappeared.

Months 5-9:   Same as Weeks 1-2

Thereafter, the woman was monitored homoeopathically and received a dose of *Natrum sulphuricum* 200c and *Scirrhinum* 200c, alternating monthly, Split Dose Method. This regimen continues to this day.

                Periodic follow-up CT scans show the liver normal.

REMARKS

Natrum sulphuricum is one of the excellent liver remedies. It was selected over *Chelidonium* because it is also an important remedy for diabetes.

Dr. Ramakrishnan's Results with Liver Cancer

	No. of Cases	No. of Viable Cases	No. of Successes	Success Rate
Pre-Plussing (<1993)	120	22	3	14%
Plussing (≥1993)	312	62	20	32%

Colon

The principal remedies for colon cancer, listed in order of frequency of use, are *Aloe, Thuja, Arsenicum album,* and *Lycopodium.*

CASE 38   *June, 1995*

Male, 55 years, presented with a diagnosed cancer of the cecum, Stage IV, which had recently been operated on.

> *History: A 6 cm. mass on the cecum was removed, together with 23 lymph glands, fifteen of which were positive for malignancy, and a hemicolectomy was performed. Chemotherapy was advised, but patient refused, turning to homoeopathy instead.*

The patient was experiencing severe cutting pains across the abdomen in the region of the transverse colon and was passing lumps of mucus, at times bloodstained—symptoms pointing to *Aloe (see Chapter 2).*

PRESCRIPTION

Week 1:   *Aloe* 200c - daily, Plussing Method

Week 2:   *Carcinosin* 200c - daily, Plussing Method

Weeks 3-8:   Same as Weeks 1-2
              Bowel movements better; no abdominal pain.

Months 3-4:   Same as Weeks 1-2, but *Aloe* in the 1M potency
              The patient gained 6 lb. and continued feeling better.

Months 5-6:   Same as Months 3-4
              The patient looked normal, felt well. Started attending to his business.

              CT scan showed clear.

Months 7-8:   Same as Months 3-4
              The patient was asymptomatic and continued feeling well.

Months 9-22:   *Aloe* 1M and *Carcinosin* 1M - alternating semi-monthly, Split Dose Method

For eighteen months longer, the patient received a dose of *Aloe* 10M or *Carcinosin* 10M , alternating monthly, Split Dose Method.

All test results continue to be normal.

CASE 39   *March, 1995*

Male, 36 years, reported with a diagnosed cancer of the colon. He was weak, emaciated, and suffered from extreme exhaustion. For the past ten years, he had been treated for ulcerative colitis with Western medicine and monitoring, until recent severe abdominal pains and rectal bleeding called for further tests.

> *Colonoscopy showed a mass in the descending colon. Biopsy revealed adenocarcinoma, Stage IIb. The patient refused surgery and chemotherapy and turned to homoeopathy instead.*

PRESCRIPTION

Week 1:   *Thuja* 200C - daily, Plussing Method

Week 2:   *Carcinosin* 200C - daily, Plussing Method

Weeks 3-16:   Same as Weeks 1-2
               The patient felt much better symptomatically. He gained 4 lb. and looked healthier. Rectal bleeding was only 25% of what it had been.

> *CT scan showed clear. Colonoscopy showed mass to be 50% of original size.*

Months 5-7:   Same as Weeks 1-2

> *Colonoscopy showed that the mass had remained at 50% of its original size.*

Months 8-11:   Same as Weeks 1-2, but in the 1M potency
               No more rectal bleeding.

> *CT scan showed clear, but patient refused to undergo any more colonoscopies, which he disliked intensely.*

Months 12-14: Same as Weeks 1-2, but in the 10M potency
By the end of this time the patient looked the picture of health and there was no recurrence of rectal bleeding. His energy was normal and he was leading an active life.

For two more years the patient was prescribed the same two remedies in the 10M potency, alternating monthly, Split Dose Method. Today he remains in good health.

CASE 40   *January, 1996*

Male, 63 years, sought homoeopathic assistance for a diagnosed cancer of the ascending colon, Stage III.

> *History: The patient had been previously treated for colon tuberculosis, which turned out to be a wrong diagnosis. A year later, colon cancer was diagnosed, and the patient turned to homoeopathy.*

The patient's personality picture was typical *Lycopodium* (see Case 27), and this remedy is a prime one for colon cancer. Thus the organ-specific remedy was obvious.

PRESCRIPTION

Week 1:   *Lycopodium* 200C† - daily, Plussing Method

Week 2:   *Carcinosin* 200C - daily, Plussing Method

Weeks 3-8:   Same as Weeks 1-2

> *CT scan not done, but upon digital examination, mass showed slight reduction in size.*

Weeks 9-16:   Same as Weeks 1-2

> *CT scan showed the mass to be the same.*

Week 17:   An abnormal gland showed up in the supraclavic-
                  ular region.

                  *It was excised and histopathology came out posi-
                  tive for cancer.*

Weeks 20-28:   Since the gland was very hard, after the operation
                  the patient was started on *Scirrhinum* 200c - daily,
                  Plussing Method.
                  He was comfortable and gained 8 lb.

Week 29:   The patient suddenly developed a profuse rectal
                  hemorrhage.

                  *He was hospitalized and a hemicolectomy was
                  performed. At the patient's insistence, no
                  chemotherapy or radiation therapy was given.*

Months 8-16 (after the operation):   Same as Weeks 1-2

                  CT scan showed everything clear.

Months 17-24: Same as Weeks 1-2, but in the 1M potency

Thereafter, the patient continued to take the two remedies, in the
1M potency, but alternating monthly, Split Dose Method—and
continues to do so to this day.

REMARKS

Scirrhinum replaced *Carcinosin* during the twentieth to twenty-
eighth weeks because the supraclavicular gland was stony hard.
But in view of subsequent events, it was thought that perhaps this
was an erroneous judgment. So after the operation, *Carcinosin*
was again resumed.

Dr. Ramakrishnan's Results with Colon Cancer

	No. of Cases	No. of Viable Cases	No. of Successes	Success Rate
Pre-Plussing (<1993)	190	63	21	33%
Plussing (≥1993)	290	70	28	40%

Rectum

The principal remedies for rectal cancer, listed in order of frequency of use, are *Nitricum acidum, Aloe, Thuja, Lachesis,* and *Sulphur.*

CASE 41   *June, 1994*

Male, 43 years, reported with alternating diarrhea and constipation for the last three months, with occasional bleeding from the rectum and recently, with more blood in the stool. He was sent for a physical examination.

> *Examination showed a hard mass, which bled on touch. A biopsy was performed; the report revealed adenocarcinoma, Stage IIa. CT scan showed no other spread.*

PRESCRIPTION

Week 1:   *Aloe* 200c - daily, Plussing Method
                  Within the first week, bleeding stopped.

Week 2:   *Scirrhinum* 200c - daily, Plussing Method

Weeks 3-16:   Same as Weeks 1-2
                  During this time, there was gradual reduction in the mass; bowel movements were normal.

Months 5-8:   Same as Weeks 1-2, but in the 1M potency

> *Examination showed the mass completely cleared.*

For six months longer, the patient received one dose of *Aloe* 1M and *Scirrhinum* 1M, alternating semimonthly, Split Dose Method.

REMARKS

For the selection of *Aloe,* see Chapter 2.

Scirrhinum, as previously noted, is the preferred nosode in rectal cancer.

CASE 42   *June, 1995*

Male, 36 years, presented with a cancer of the rectum, with needling, splinter-like pains.

> *Biopsy revealed an adenocarcinoma, Stage II. CT scan was clear with regard to abdominal organs— no metastasis.*

Over the past twenty years, the patient had been subject to various lesions in the rectum and several times had been operated on for hemorrhoids and fissures in the anus. The type of pain, recurrent episodes of stomatitis, and an intense desire for salt and fatty foods all pointed to *Nitricum acidum*.

PRESCRIPTION

Week 1:   *Nitricum acidum* 200C - daily, Plussing Method

Week 2:   *Scirrhinum* 200C - daily, Plussing Method

Weeks 3-12:   Same as Weeks 1-2

> *The lesion was examined by his surgeon, who pronounced it to be significantly reduced in size.*

Months 4-6:   Same as Weeks 1-2

> *Lesion had completely healed.*

Month 7:   *Nitricum acidum* 1M - semimonthly, Split Dose Method

Month 8:   *Scirrhinum* 1M - semimonthly, Split Dose Method

Months 9-12:   Same as Months 7-8

End of treatment. The patient is monitored and continues perfectly healthy.

CASE 43 [p-P]   *November, 1988*

Male, 53 years, had a mass in the rectum almost at the anal margin, which bled at the slightest touch. There was also a pricking pain as if with needles.

> *Biopsy revealed a squamous cell carcinoma,*
> *Stage II.*

The patient was irritable, headstrong, with a craving for salt and fried foods, and all symptoms were ameliorated when traveling (whether in a car, airplane, or train)—in short, a typical *Nitricum acidum* personality type. There was a family history of tuberculosis.

PRESCRIPTION

Weeks 1-4:   *Nitricum acidum* 200c† - weekly, Split Dose
               Method
               The patient felt only slightly better.

Weeks 5-6:   *Sulphur* 200c - weekly, Split Dose Method
               Again, the patient felt only slightly better.

Week 7:   *Tuberculinum bovinum* 200c - weekly, Split Dose
               Method
               No noticeable marked improvement.

Weeks 8-10:   *Sulphur* 200c - weekly, Split Dose Method
               Mass was less than 50% of its original size.

               A profuse hemorrhage during this time necessitat-
               ed some local allopathic medication and dressing.

Weeks 12-16:   *Nitricum acidum* 200c - weekly, Split Dose
               Method

Weeks 17-21:   *Carcinosin* 200c - weekly, Split Dose Method
               Another significant reduction in size of the mass.

Weeks 22-72:   *Nitricum acidum* 200c and *Carcinosin* 200c, alter-
               nating weekly, Split Dose Method
               Improvement continued.

Months 18-30: Same as Weeks 22-72, but in the 1M potency
Upon examination, the mass was seen to be 10% of its original size.

Thereafter, and to this day, the patient receives periodic doses of either *Nitricum acidum* 1M or *Carcinosin* 1M. The final outcome is that the mass remains 10% of its original size—a flat ulceration, slightly raised and about ½ inch in diameter. For twelve years now the patient has been comfortable and leading a normal life. The lesion is 100% localized, with no spread whatsoever.

REMARKS

Sulphur was prescribed because the desired result was not forthcoming, and it seemed necessary to shift to another remedy effective for rectal cancer.

Likewise, *Tuberculinum bovinum* was prescribed to obtain better results—and the remedy seemed the most appropriate nosode in view of the history of tuberculosis in the patient's family. Also, one recalls that in the earlier days, Dr. Ramakrishnan was not as convinced of the prime importance of *Carcinosin* and *Scirrhinum,* and he was still experimenting with the different nosodes. (See also Cases 7, 62, 77, and 95.)

Finally, *Nitricum acidum* was reintroduced to give the seemingly "most similar remedy" another try. Since the patient was stable and doing well by 1993, Dr. Ramakrishnan judged it best not to rock the boat, but continue with the same treatment. Hence no Plussing Method was used.

For an additional example of successful treatment of this type of cancer, see Case 99.

DR. RAMAKRISHNAN'S RESULTS WITH RECTAL CANCER

	No. of Cases	No. of Viable Cases	No. of Successes	Success Rate
Pre-Plussing (<1993)	50	26	18	69%
Plussing (≥1993)	170	66	54	82%

Bladder

The principal remedies for bladder cancer, listed in order of frequency of use, are *Terebinthina, Thuja,* and *Conium.*

CASE 44 [p-P]   *March, 1990*

Male, 24 years, presented with blood in the urine and burning for the past three weeks.

> *Cystoscopy revealed a 2.5 cm. ulcer on the bladder wall. Biopsy report: squamous cell carcinoma, Stage II. No other glandular or metastatic involvement.*

PRESCRIPTION

Week 1:   *Terebinthina* 200c - daily, Split Dose Method

Week 2:   *Carcinosin* 200c - daily, Split Dose Method
                Bleeding and burning stopped 10 days after treatment was initiated. The patient was comfortable.

Weeks 3-12:   Same as Weeks 1-2

> *Cystoscopy showed the lesion healed more than 50%.*

Months 4-6:   Same as Weeks 1-2, but in the 1M potency

> *Cystoscopy showed a further 20% to 25% reduction in size.*

Months 7-9:   Same as Months 4-6

> *Cystoscopy showed that total reduction of lesion remained at 75%.*

Months 10-16:   Same as Months 4-6, but in the 10M potency

Thereafter, the patient would periodically receive a constitutional remedy or *Carcinosin* 1M, and his condition has remained stable.

No further cystoscopies or scans have been per-
formed because the patient, feeling well, refused
(and still refuses) to go for further tests. Hence
there is no information about further reduction of
the size of the lesion.

CASE 45   *December, 1994*

Male, 53 years, was experiencing repeated blood in the urine.

Cystoscopy and biopsy revealed a cauliflower
growth, which was diagnosed as an adeno-
carcinoma, Stage II.

The patient was sensitive to cold, disliked raw onions because they brought on insomnia, had suffered from asthma since childhood, and had numerous moles on different parts of his body—all typical of *Thuja*.

PRESCRIPTION

Week 1:   *Thuja* 200c† - daily, Plussing Method

Week 2:   *Carcinosin* 200c - daily, Plussing Method

Weeks 3-8:   Same as Weeks 1-2
               Bleeding stopped.

               CT scan showed the growth smaller in size. No
               metastasis.

Months 3-4:   Same as Weeks 1-2

               CT scan showed growth further reduced in size.

Months 5-8:   Same as Weeks 1-2, but in the 1M potency

               CT scan showed mass completely gone.

Months 9-11:   Same as Weeks 1-2, but in the 10M potency

For six months longer, *Thuja* 10M and *Carcinosin* 10M were prescribed, alternating semimonthly, Split Dose Method.

REMARKS

Thuja was prescribed for the patient's constitutional type and because of its prominent role as an organ-specific remedy in the treatment of cancers of the genitourinary system.

For an additional example of successful treatment of this type of cancer, see Case 101.

Dr. Ramakrishnan's Results with Cancer of the Bladder

	No. of Cases	No. of Viable Cases	No. of Successes	Success Rate
Pre-Plussing (<1993)	46	18	10	56%
Plussing (≥1993)	94	36	26	72%

Prostate

The principal remedies for prostate cancer, listed in order of frequency of use, are *Thuja, Conium, Sabal serrulata,* and *Lycopodium.*

CASE 46   *May, 1996*

Male, 58 years, presented with secondary nodes in the presacral area and deposits in the liver (picked up by a CT scan). His PSA was 13.3.

> *History: January, 1995, adenocarcinoma of the median lobe of prostate was diagnosed, Stage IIb. The entire prostate and testicles were removed, followed by radiation therapy.*

The patient had deep lines on his face; he was intellectual, with a caustic wit, and every day felt sleepy around 5:00 p.m.

PRESCRIPTION

Week 1:	*Conium* 200C - daily, Plussing Method
Week 2:	*Scirrhinum* 200C - daily, Plussing Method
Weeks 3-8:	Same as Weeks 1-2

> *No change was seen in scan, but his PSA dropped to 7.5.*

Weeks 9-16:	Same as Weeks 1-2

> *Test showed presacral nodes 80% reduced; PSA 4.2. Deposits in the liver unchanged.*

Week 17:	*Lycopodium* 200C† - daily, Plussing Method
Week 18:	*Scirrhinum* 200C - daily, Plussing Method
Weeks 19-24:	Same as Weeks 17-18

> *Tests showed deposits in liver decreased by 25%. PSA still at 4.2.*

Months 7-9:	Same as Weeks 17-18, but in the 1M potency.

*CT scan showed nodes and deposits to be almost
entirely gone; PSA down to 3.2.*

For eighteen months, the patient received *Lycopodium* 1M and *Scirrhinum* 1M , alternating semimonthly, Split Dose Method. Today he is active, asymptomatic, and comfortable—and his condition has remained stable.

*Subsequent six-monthly CT scans and assays of
PSA level showed everything the same as the
Month 9 test results.*

REMARKS

Scirrhinum, as was noted earlier, is often the preferred nosode in prostate cancer because usually the gland is very hard.

Lycopodium was selected because it is a prominent prostate remedy and it fit the patient's constitutional type.

CASE 47   *May, 1996*

Male, 49 years, presented with a history of prostate cancer, which had been operated on (a 1 cm. × 7 cm. nodule in the presacral region and a 0.5 cm. × 1 cm. nodule in the left supraclavicular area had been excised), followed by radiation therapy. A scan had showed surrounding organs and bones clear. But a later MRI showed a return of the cancer.

*The pathology report on the supraclavicular gland
was positive for malignancy, and the opinion of the
oncologist, after an MRI of the presacral region,
was that it was a metastasized lymph node, Stage I.*

There was a strong history of cancer in the patient's family.

PRESCRIPTION

Week 1:   *Conium* 200C - daily, Plussing Method

Week 2:   *Carcinosin* 200C - daily, Plussing Method

Weeks 3-12:   Same as Weeks 1-2

MRI showed the metastatic gland in the presacral region was 50% reduced.

Months 4-6:   Same as Weeks 1-2

CT scan and bone scan of his entire body showed the presacral lymph node normal and the whole body clear.

For twelve more months, *Conium* 1M and *Carcinosin* 1M, alternating monthly, Split Dose Method, were given.

Thereafter, no more medication—and the patient continues well.

REMARKS

In this case, *Carcinosin* was selected rather than *Scirrhinum* (as in Cases 46 and 48) because of the family history of cancer *(see Chapters 2 and 9).*

CASE 48   *May, 1994*

Male, 58 years, presented with a diagnosed prostate cancer. Symptoms were burning during urination and impeded flow.

Biopsy report: Squamous cell carcinoma, Stage II.

The patient had had several bouts with sexually transmitted diseases: herpes, gonorrhea, etc., as well as recurring cystitis and prostatitis.

PRESCRIPTION

Week 1:   *Sabal serrulata* 200c - daily, Plussing Method

Week 2:   *Scirrhinum* 200c - daily, Plussing Method

Weeks 3-4:   Same as Weeks 1-2
               Urinary symptoms better: no burning and flow improved.

Months 2-4:   Same as Weeks 1-2

> *On rectal examination a tumor could no longer be discerned, and a CT scan indicated prostate was near-normal in size.*

Months 5-8:   Same as Weeks 1-2, but in the 1M potency

> *As far as could be ascertained from tests and palpation prostate was normal in size.*

Months 9-20:   Same two remedies in the 1M potency, alternating monthly, Split Dose Method.

> *Periodic examinations during this time confirmed no sign of tumor.*

For one more year, same as Months 9-20, but in the 1M potency.

REMARKS

Recurrent sexually transmitted diseases suggest *Sabal serrulata*. Also, *Sabal* was given instead of *Conium* because the gland did not feel hard; it was more nodular and fairly soft.

For additional examples of successful treatment of this type of cancer, see Cases 1, 111, and 112.

DR. RAMAKRISHNAN'S RESULTS WITH PROSTATE CANCER

	No. of Cases	No. of Viable Cases	No. of Successes	Success Rate
Pre-Plussing (<1993)	80	51	24	47%
Plussing (≥1993)	150	90	72	80%

Ovary

The principal remedies for ovarian cancer, listed in order of frequency of use, are *Aurum muriaticum natronatum, Viburnum prunifolium, Thuja, Sepia,* and *Lilium tigrinum.*

CASE 49   *January, 1996*

Female, 32 years, reported with diagnosed cancerous secondary glands in the pelvis and abdomen, following in the wake of a primary ovarian cancer.

> *History: In 1995, a CT scan and laparoscopic biopsy confirmed squamous cell carcinoma, with fixed secondaries in pelvic and abdominal areas, Stage III. The patient was operated on, but the glands could not be removed. Chemotherapy and radiation therapy were advised, but patient refused and turned to homoeopathy instead.*

The woman was active, impulsive (everything had to be done in a hurry), with increased sexual desire. Physically she was experiencing a bearing-down sensation in the uterine region and some bloating. Her entire picture fit *Lilium tigrinum* well.

PRESCRIPTION

Week 1:	*Lilium tigrinum* 200C† - daily, Plussing Method
Week 2:	*Carcinosin* 200C - daily, Plussing Method
Weeks 3-8:	Same as Weeks 1-2 Everything was stable.
Months 3-4:	Same as Weeks 1-2

> *MRI showed significant reduction in the size of the glands.*

Months 5-6:	Same as Weeks 1-2, but in the 1M potency

CT scan and other tests since commencement of treatment revealed all the secondary deposits to have shrunk considerably—more than 50%.

Months 7-12:   Same as Months 5-6

CT scan showed the ovary cleared of lesion; and showed secondary glands further reduced.

Months 13-17: Same as Months 5-6

Further tests showed everything clear.

For one year, *Lilium tigrinum* 1M and *Carcinosin* 1M were prescribed, alternating semimonthly, Split Dose Method. Thereafter, the woman received periodic doses of either *Lilium tigrinum* 1M or *Carcinosin* 1M. She continues to do well symptomatically.

REMARKS

Lilium tigrinum, apart from fitting the patient's symptom picture, is one of the best remedies for cancers of the female reproductive organs *(see Chapter 2).*

CASE 50   *June, 1995*

Female, 44 years, presented with a diagnosed malignant cyst of the right ovary, Stage II.

The patient had refused recommended surgery and chemotherapy and had opted for homoeopathy instead.

The woman was weepy, apt to complain, indifferent to her loved ones, and striving for independence—all typical *Sepia* mental symptoms.

PRESCRIPTION

Week 1:   *Sepia* 200c† - daily, Plussing Method

Week 2:   *Carcinosin* 200c - daily, Plussing Method

Weeks 3-8:   Same as Weeks 1-2

Tests showed a 50% reduction of the cyst's original size.

Months 3-4:   Same as Weeks 1-2
Not much observable change.

Months 5-6:   Same as Weeks 1-2, but in the 1M potency

Tests showed that the mass was reduced to 10% of its original size.

Months 7-9:   Same as Months 5-6

Tests showed mass unchanged.

At this point the woman refused to continue the Plussing Method, and for the next year, she received the two remedies in the 1M potency—alternating weekly, Split Dose Method. Thereafter, the remedies were given only occasionally, as her symptoms and mood dictated.

The mass remains at 10% of its original size.

REMARKS

Apart from fitting the patient's constitutional picture, *Sepia* is a prominent remedy for cancerous affections of the female reproductive system *(see Chapter 2)*.

For additional examples of successful treatment of this type of cancer, see Cases 6, 109, 110, 119, and 120.

Dr. Ramakrishnan's Results with Ovarian Cancer

	No. of Cases	No. of Viable Cases	No. of Successes	Success Rate
Pre-Plussing (<1993)	65	20	11	55%
Plussing (≥1993)	95	35	24	69%

Uterus

The principal remedies for uterine cancer, listed in order of frequency of use, are *Aurum muriaticum natronatum, Thuja, Sepia, Viburnum prunifolium, Lachesis,* and *Lilium tigrinum.*

CASE 51   *February, 1996*

Female, 52 years, presented with uterine cancer. For many months she had been experiencing a severe hip pain radiating down to the thigh.

> *History: After three years of no menstrual periods, the patient experienced periodic vaginal bleeding. After a year, she visited a gynecologist who performed a D&C. Tests revealed adenocarcinoma of the uterus, Stage III. The patient turned down the insistent advice of an immediate hysterectomy and chose homoeopathy instead.*

Physically, the woman had a history of thick, profuse, greenish leucorrhea until menopause (four years earlier), and for twenty years multiple warts in the vulval region. In her personality picture, she was impressionable, artistic (a born actress), somewhat flighty by nature and irresponsible, but always well-meaning.

PRESCRIPTION

Week 1:   *Thuja* 200c - daily, Plussing Method

Week 2:   *Scirrhinum* 200c - daily, Plussing Method

Weeks 3-4:   Same as Weeks 1-2
               The patient felt better overall, but there was not much change in the bleeding.

Weeks 5-8:   Same as Weeks 1-2
               The patient bled less. The hip pain was considerably better.

Weeks 9-16:   Same as Weeks 1-2, but in the 1M potency
               The vaginal bleeding stopped completely.

> *CT scan showed no involvement of nearby organs
> or any metastatic glands.*

Weeks 17-18:   Same as Weeks 1-2, but in the 1M potency.
               The patient was totally symptom free.

Weeks 19-36:   Same as Weeks 17-18

Thereafter, the woman received *Thuja* 10M or *Scirrhinum* 10M, alternating monthly, Split Dose Method. This regimen continues to this day. The patient is periodically strongly urged to go for a D&C to ascertain the state of the uterus, but she refuses to do so. Almost five years later, she is still in good health, and the warts she had for twenty years have disappeared.

REMARKS

Thuja is well-known for genital warts and thick, greenish, profuse mucous discharges. It is also, as was noted earlier, one of the primary remedies for cancers of the male and female reproductive organs.

Scirrhinum was selected over *Carcinosin* because of the woman's highly *Phosphorus* personality type (see Remarks in Case 4).

CASE 52   *January, 1996*

Female, 63 years, presented with off-and-on vaginal bleeding for the last year. Since it was not profuse, she did not bother to see a specialist. When she did, she was diagnosed with an adenocarcinoma of the uterus.

> *Internal examination and ultrasound showed a
> mass 4 cm. in diameter; CT scan and biopsy con-
> firmed an adenocarcinoma, Stage III.*

Seeking to avoid surgery, chemotherapy, or radiation therapy, the woman turned to homoeopathy. She was loquacious, exuded plentiful vitality, and had always experienced relief of her premenstrual symptoms once the flow set in—all characteristics pointing to *Lachesis*.

PRESCRIPTION

Week 1:	*Aurum muriaticum natronatum* 200C - daily, Plussing Method
Week 2:	*Scirrhinum* 200C - daily, Plussing Method
Weeks 3-20:	Same as Weeks 1-2

> *Internal examination and CT scan showed mass to be smaller by 15% to 20%.*

Months 6-9:   Same as Weeks 1-2, but in the 1M potency
Symptomatically she was free of bleeding, or even spotting; had gained 8 lb. and looked healthy.

> *Mass was reduced by another 10%.*

Months 10-13: Same as Months 6-9

> *No change in size of mass.*

Months 14-18: Same as Weeks 1-2, but in the 10M potency

> *Still no change in mass size.*

Months 19-26: *Lachesis* 10M† and *Scirrhinum* 10M, alternating weekly - daily, Plussing Method

> *CT scan showed no change and no metastasis.*

Thereafter, the woman was put on a maintenance regimen—alternating monthly doses of *Aurum muriaticum natronatum* 10M and *Scirrhinum* 10M, Split Dose Method. She remains well to date.

REMARKS

Aurum muriaticum natronatum was selected to open the case because of its preeminent role in uterine cancer. It was returned to after *Lachesis* surprisingly brought about no marked improvement.

Also, see the last paragraph in Chapter 8.

Dr. Ramakrishnan's Results with Uterine Cancer

	No. of Cases	No. of Viable Cases	No. of Successes	Success Rate
Pre-Plussing (<1993)	90	24	6	25%
Plussing (≥1993)	120	33	15	45%

Cervix

The principal remedies for cervical cancer, listed in order of frequency of use, are *Aurum muriaticum natronatum, Pulsatilla, Sepia,* and *Lilium tigrinum.*

CASE 53   *June, 1995*

Female, 39 years, reported with a leucorrhea of many years standing, which was now accompanied by severe pulling pains all over the hypogastrium and lumbosacral region. These would come on suddenly, but decrease only gradually—and were more pronounced in the evening.

> *Examination showed ulcer on cervix and biopsy report confirmed squamous cell carcinoma, Stage II.*

The patient was gentle, soft spoken, sensitive, affectionate; worse from rich, fatty foods; better from a breeze and gentle (rather than vigorous) exercise—in a word, a classic *Pulsatilla.*

PRESCRIPTION

Week 1:	*Pulsatilla* 200c - daily, Plussing Method
Week 2:	*Carcinosin* 200c - daily, Plussing Method
Weeks 3-8:	Same as Weeks 1-2 Leucorrhea stopped.
Months 3-4:	Same as Weeks 1-2, but in the 1M potency The ulcer was healing, with less bleeding and pain.
Months 5-6:	Same as Months 3-4 Cervical lesion 90% cured.
Months 7-8:	Same as Months 3-4 The patient was clear of all symptoms.

> *All tests and examinations showed normal.*

After this, for twelve months, the woman received *Pulsatilla* 10M and *Carcinosin* 10M, alternating monthly, Split Dose Method.

End of treatment.

REMARKS

As can be observed from the ovarian, uterine, and cervical cancer cases cited, when prescribing for the female reproductive organs, one tends to individualize more—employing the classical "female" constitutional remedies, such as *Sepia, Pulsatilla, Lilium tigrinum,* and *Lachesis.*

CASE 54   *November, 1995*

Female, 63 years, fifteen years after menopause, was experiencing vaginal bleeding.

> *Examination revealed an ulcer on cervix and biopsy reported squamous cell carcinoma, Stage IIb.*

The woman, *Sepia*-like, was strong-willed, hardworking; often feeling injured or depressed and wanting to be left alone. During her entire married life, she had had little or no inclination for marital relations.

PRESCRIPTION

Week 1:	*Sepia* 200 c† - daily, Plussing Method
Week 2:	*Carcinosin* 200c - daily, Plussing Method
Weeks 3-8:	Same as Weeks 1-2 Ulcer looked only marginally better, but patient felt much healthier and more cheerful.
Months 3-4:	Same as Weeks 1-2 Ulcer had shrunk 30% to 40%. No bleeding, no discharge.

Months 5-6:   Same as Weeks 1-2, but in the 1M potency
               The patient reported additional progress in ener-
               gy and mood.

Months 7-8:   Same as Months 5-6
               Ulcer fully healed.

               CT scan of abdominal cavity showed all organs
               clear.

Months 9-12:   Same as Months 5-6

For an additional eight months, the woman received the two
remedies in the 10M potency, alternating monthly, Split Dose
Method.

REMARKS

See Remarks in Case 53.

CASE 55   *April, 1994*

Female, 41 years, presented with a malignant ulcer on the cervix
and a mass on right ovary. She had leucorrhea, bleeding, and
burning in uterus.

Examination and tests reported a metastatic lesion
from the cervix, Stage III.

The woman was experiencing a bearing-down sensation in uterus
and increased sexual desire; she was also oversensitive and extremely high-strung.

PRESCRIPTION

Week 1:   *Lilium tigrinum* 200C† - daily, Plussing Method

Week 2:   *Carcinosin* 200C - daily, Plussing Method

Weeks 3-8:   Same as Weeks 1-2

> *Physical palpation indicated that the ovarian mass had completely disappeared. This was confirmed by CT scan.*

Months 3-4:   Same as Weeks 1-2
Symptoms of bleeding, burning, and bearing-down sensation were all better.

Ulcer looked better.

Months 5-6:   Same as Weeks 1-2, but in the 1M potency
No symptoms whatsoever.

Ulcer had shrunk to 75%.

Months 7-12:   Same as Months 5-6

Ulcer had shrunk even further and was down to 30%.

Months 13-18:   Same as Months 5-6

Ulcer had not changed.

Months 19-24:   Same two remedies, but in the 10M potency, alternating semimonthly, Split Dose Method

Ulcer not changed.

Thereafter, although semiyearly gynecological examinations showed that ulcer had never completely healed, the condition remains stable and the patient healthy and asymptomatic.

REMARKS

See Remarks in Case 53.

For an additional example of successful treatment of this type of cancer, see Case 3.

Dr. Ramakrishnan's Results with Cervical Cancer

	No. of Cases	No. of Viable Cases	No. of Successes	Success Rate
Pre-Plussing (<1993)	80	26	10	38%
Plussing (≥1993)	104	44	30	68%

Bone

The principal remedies for bone cancer (including myeloma, sarcoma, osteoclastoma, Ewing's sarcoma, etc.), listed in order of frequency of use, are *Hekla lava, Symphytum, Aurum metallicum,* and *Calcarea carbonica.*

CASE 56   *November, 1995*

Male, 54 years, presented with a diagnosed myeloma, Stage II. There was a swelling over the fourth rib; otherwise patient was asymptomatic.

> *CT scan showed a lytic lesion in fourth rib and multiple small lesions in other ribs and vertebrae.*

The patient admitted to anticipatory and other anxieties; he was fond of people but felt claustrophobic in crowds. Physically, he had a craving for sweets, which, however, disagreed with him, and he was subject to occasional sharp, painful spasms in the muscles of the chest. These symptoms pointed to *Argentum nitricum.*

PRESCRIPTION

Week 1:   *Argentum nitricum* 200C† - daily, Plussing Method

Week 2:   *Hekla lava* 200C - daily, Plussing Method

Weeks 3-4:   Same as Weeks 1-2
               The swelling on the right rib was reduced from its original size by 25%.

Month 2:   Same as Weeks 1-2
               Further improvement was visible.

Month 3:   Same as Weeks 1-2

               CT scan showed lytic lesion on rib 75% reduced and other multiple lesions completely cleared. Hematology report showed plasma cells considerably reduced.

Months 4-8:   Same as Weeks 1-2, but in the 1M potency

All tests showed ribs and vertebrae completely clear.

Month 9:   The patient was going on a vacation and sought permission to take a month's rest from the Plussing Method. Because he was doing well, permission was granted.

Months 10-13:   Same as Month 8

Thereafter, and to date, single doses of *Argentum nitricum* 1M and *Hekla lava* 1M, alternating monthly, Split Dose Method, were prescribed.

REMARKS

This is a rare example of a post-1993 case where Dr. Ramakrishnan did not use any cancer nosode. *Hekla lava* obviated this necessity.

CASE 57   *May, 1995*

Male, 62 years, was experiencing intolerable pain in chest; also in specific spots, all over the body. He had been diagnosed as having myeloma, Stage III.

Bone scan revealed multiple spots of increased radio uptake all over skeletal system, but especially around ribs and vertebrae. Biopsy report was positive for plasmatic myeloma. Plasma cells 42%, normoblasts 12%, paraprotein mononuclear cells (PMN) 16%, myelocytes 5%, metamyelocytes 1%, megakaryocytes 1%.

PRESCRIPTION

Week 1:   *Hekla lava* 200c - daily, Plussing Method

Week 2:   *Carcinosin* 200c - daily, Plussing Method
Some relief from pain.

Weeks 3-4:   Same as Weeks 1-2
               Great relief from pain.

Months 2-5:   Same as Weeks 1-2
               The patient was now very comfortable.

               Blood tests showed improvement.

Months 6-8:   Same as Weeks 1-2, but in the 1M potency

               *Bone scan showed nearly 50% of the deposits
               cleared.*

Months 9-12:   Same as Months 6-8

               *Bone marrow aspiration showed plasma cell 10%,
               normoblasts 2%, and no metamyelocytes or
               megakaryocytes.*

Months 13-18: Same two remedies in the 1M potency, alternating
               weekly, Split Dose Method

Thereafter, the patient reported regularly and received a dose of
Hekla lava 1M or *Carcinosin* 1M, alternating monthly, Split Dose
Method.

REMARKS

Hekla lava's extraordinary healing power in cancers of the bone
requires no elaboration.

CASE 58   *October, 1995*

Male, 68 years, reported to his homoeopath after a recent bone
scan revealed secondary deposits in the pelvic and lower lumbar
region, Stage III. What prompted the scan was excruciating pain
in his right hip: a gnawing sensation, or like driving a screw into
the bone.

*History: Prostatic cancer operated on and followed
by radiation therapy in 1993. After the bone scan
revealed new deposits, radiation therapy was again*

suggested. The patient refused and turned to homoeopathy instead.

PRESCRIPTION

Week 1:   *Aurum metallicum* 200c - daily, Plussing Method

Week 2:   *Carcinosin* 200c - daily, Plussing Method
The patient reported a slight reduction of the pain.

Weeks 3-8:   Same as Weeks 1-2
The patient reported further reduction of the pain.

Months 3-4:   Same as Weeks 1-2
The patient continued to feel better.

Bone scan showed deposits to be less.

Months 5-8:   Same as Weeks 1-2, but in the 1M potency
The pain was almost entirely gone.

Scan revealed 80% to 90% clearance of deposits.

Months 9-12:   Same as Months 5-8
The patient had fully recovered.

Scan revealed clearance of all deposits.

Thereafter, and for the next six months, the patient received *Aurum metallicum* 1M and *Carcinosin* 1M, alternating semimonthly, Split Dose Method. Then he stopped treatment on his own. He continues well to date.

REMARKS

For severe bone pains in cancerous affections, *Aurum metallicum* has few equals.

For additional examples of successful treatment of this type of cancer, see Cases 95, 96, and 121.

Dr. Ramakrishnan's Results with Bone Cancer

	No. of Cases	No. of Viable Cases	No. of Successes	Success Rate
Pre-Plussing (<1993)	76	22	10	45%
Plussing (≥1993)	114	42	31	74%

Leukemia

The principal remedies for leukemia, listed in order of frequency of use, are *Hekla lava, Symphytum, Ceanothus americanus*, and *Strontia*.

CASE 59   *September, 1997*

Female child, 1½ years, presented with diagnosed acute lymphoid leukemia, Stage II.

> *Cytochemistry showed blast cells, black fine granules seen. Hemoglobin down to 2.5 gm./dL. Platelet count 6000. Blood transfusion given. After transfer, hemoglobin 3.4 gm./dL., platelets 20,000.*

PRESCRIPTION

Week 1:   *Hekla lava* 200c - daily, Plussing Method

Week 2:   *Carcinosin* 200c - daily, Plussing Method
              Child looked healthier and was more cheerful.

Weeks 3-4:   Same as Weeks 1-2
              Improvement maintained.

Month 2:   Same as Weeks 1-2
              Condition further improved.

Months 3-4:   Same as Weeks 1-2, but in the 1M potency
              Child looked perfectly normal.

> *Blood smear: No blast cells, no atypical cells, hemoglobin 10.3 gm./dL., platelets 90,000.*

Months 5-9:   Same as Months 3-4, but weekly, Split Dose Method

Thereafter, the child was seen once a month and was (and still is) prescribed for constitutionally—usually *Pulsatilla* or *Tuberculinum (see Chapter 7)*. She is perfectly healthy.

REMARKS

Once again one observes the sovereign role of *Hekla lava* in the treatment of cancers of the bone and bone marrow.

N.B. With children, once their cancer has been helped, one usually does not have to continue as long with the Plussing or weekly Split Dose Method as with adults (see Cases 9, 10, 60, 62, and 96).

CASE 60   *May, 1993*

Male child, 6 years, was brought in with chronic myelogenous leukemia, Stage II. A large number of glands were affected, which were unusually hard for chronic myelogenous leukemia. The boy was febrile, and had an enlarged liver and spleen. He was also thirstless and had an oedematous face.

PRESCRIPTION

Week 1:   *Apis* 200c - daily, Plussing Method

Week 2:   *Scirrhinum* 200c - daily, Plussing Method

Weeks 3-4:   Same as Weeks 1-2
               Glands were less hard, no new glands appeared to be affected, and the periodic fevers were much reduced.

               Hemoglobin count had risen from 6.5 to 8 gm./dL.

Months 2-3:   Same as Weeks 1-2

               Child was afebrile and glands were reduced in size by 25%. Liver and spleen also much reduced in size, but the leukemic blood picture was unchanged.

Months 4-7:   *Symphytum* 200c and *Scirrhinum* 200c, alternating weekly - daily, Plussing Method

               Blood test results were completely normal.

Months 8-12: *Symphytum* 200c and *Scirrhinum* 200c, alternating monthly, Split Dose Method

> *In this case, a CT scan of the liver and spleen was done every three months. The last two, in months nine and twelve, came out completely normal—no sign of enlargement of liver or spleen.*

For one year longer, the child continued to receive the same as Months 8-12, but in the 1M potency. After that, only occasional remedies were given as needed.

REMARKS

Apis is one of the first remedies to consider when there is oedema in the picture.

Scirrhinum was prescribed because of the unusual hardness of the affected glands.

Symphytum was prescribed rather than *Hekla lava* because of the history of periodic bouts with inflammation of the joints and arthralgia *(see Chapter 2)*.

CASE 61   *November, 1995*

Female, 37 years, sought homoeopathic assistance for recurrent small, hard lumps cropping up around the supraclavicular and submandibular areas of her body. No fevers.

> *History: The patient had been operated on for non-Hodgkin's lymphoma, followed by chemotherapy, less than a year earlier. Recent bone marrow aspiration report confirmed non-Hodgkin's lymphoma, Stage IV.*

The woman suffered from periodic digestive problems, including nausea at the sight, smell, or even thought of food; also constipation. By nature she was independent, hard-working, liked her job as an interior decorator, and took pride in being unsentimental and unemotional.

PRESCRIPTION

Week 1:   *Hekla lava* 200c - daily, Plussing Method

Week 2:   *Scirrhinum* 200c - daily, Plussing Method

Weeks 3-4:   Same as Weeks 1-2
               A gradual reduction in size of lumps was notice-
               able.

Months 2-3:   Same as Weeks 1-2
               The gradual but satisfactory reduction in size
               continued.

Months 4-6:   Same as Weeks 1-2, but in the 1M potency
               Improvement continued—almost no signs of
               lymphomas.

               *Once a month the entire blood work was repeated
               and it showed steady, all-around improvement.*

Months 7-9:   Same as Months 4-6

               Blood work showed continued improvement.

               At this point, Dr. Ramakrishnan judged it time for
               the constitutional remedy.

Months 10-12: *Sepia* 200c† - weekly, Split Dose Method
               Lymphomas all disappeared.

Months 13-15: Same as Months 10-12

Thereafter, and to date, the woman has been receiving *Hekla lava*
1M, *Scirrhinum* 1M, or Sepia 1M, once a month, Split Dose
Method. There has been no recurrence.

REMARKS

This case exemplifies how, once improvement has clearly set in,
the prescriber can move on to the constitutional remedy if he sees
a distinct picture *(see Chapter 7).*

CASE 62 [p-P]   *September, 1989*

Male child, 3 years, was brought in with myelogenous leukemia, Stage II. He had been having recurrent fevers since April, 1989, and had been growing disproportionately weak. Spleen slightly enlarged.

Blood tests showed hemoglobin count to be 8.6 gm./dL.; bone marrow study confirmed leukemia. Blast cells elevated, megakaryocytes 6, platelets 30,000. The patient's parents decided to try homoeopathic treatment first, before they would consider the chemotherapeutic drug suggested by the hematologist.

The boy had a history of tuberculosis at 1½ years of age, for which he was treated for nine months. He was, constitutionally, a *Silica:* shy, timid, sensitive; physically delicate, with a milk intolerance and prone to ear discharges that were watery, bloody, and offensive smelling; and to infections that were slow to heal.

PRESCRIPTION

Weeks 1-4:   *Ceanothus americanus* 200c - weekly, Split Dose Method

Week 5:   *Tuberculinum bovinum* 200c - weekly, Split Dose Method
              Child looked brighter, less pale.

              Hemoglobin rose to 9 gm./dL.

Weeks 6-9:   Same as Week 1
              Child was clinically better. No fevers.

              Platelet count went up from 30,000 to 45,000.

Week 10:   Suddenly child took a turn for the worse.

              Hemoglobin 4.6 gm./dL., platelets down to 20,000, blood transfusion given. Steroid medications and chemotherapy were advised. The patient's parents resisted.

Weeks 11-14: *Tuberculinum bovinum* 200c - weekly, Split Dose Method
Remarkable improvement.

Weeks 15-18: *Silica* 200c† - weekly, Split Dose Method
Child continued to improve.

Weeks 19-34: *Tuberculinum bovinum* 200c and *Silica* 200c - given weekly, Split Dose Method, alternating remedies every four weeks
Child made a complete recovery. Spleen was back to normal size.

No blast cells; no megakaryocytes. Yearly blood pictures show everything normal to date.

Thereafter, periodic constitutional remedies have kept the boy healthy.

REMARKS

Ceanothus americanus, an excellent remedy for anemia, is also one of the best remedies for leukemia. It was selected over *Hekla lava* because of the splenetic enlargement; the remedy is highly specific to the spleen *(see Chapter 2).*

Tuberculinum was the preferred nosode because of the child's history of tuberculosis (see also Remarks in Case 43).

DR. RAMAKRISHNAN'S RESULTS WITH LEUKEMIA

	No. of Cases	No. of Viable Cases	No. of Successes	Success Rate
Pre-Plussing (<1993)	115	40	12	30%
Plussing (≥1993)	205	65	35	54%

Hodgkin's Lymphoma

The principal remedies for Hodgkin's lymphoma, listed in order of frequency of use, are *Aurum metallicum, Iodum, Spongia, Scrophularia nodosa*, and *Thuja*.

CASE 63   *May, 1996*

Female, 32 years, had noticed two or three swollen glands in the left cervical region, a temperature rise every night, and night sweats. Within another ten days, two more soft, rubbery, or spongy glands appeared in the left inguinal region. The patient was sent for a biopsy.

> *Biopsy on cervical gland came out as Hodgkin's lymphoma. Since spleen was also enlarged, it was assessed as Stage III and chemotherapy was advised. The patient refused and opted for homoeopathy.*

PRESCRIPTION

Week 1:	*Spongia* 200c - daily, Plussing Method
Week 2:	*Carcinosin* 200c - daily, Plussing Method Only occasional fever spikes and temperature less elevated.
Weeks 3-4:	Same as Weeks 1-2 During this time, fever had steadily come down and become normal. No change in the glands or spleen enlargement.
Months 2-4:	Same as Weeks 1-2 Significant reduction in the size of the glands. *CT scan showed reduction in the size of the spleen.*
Months 5-6:	Same as Weeks 1-2, but both remedies raised to the 1M potency Glands were almost normal size.

CT scan showed spleen and abdominal organs, including liver, as normal.

Months 7-12:   Same as Months 5-6
Glands completely normal and the patient was doing well all this time.

Months 13-24: Same remedies in the 1M potency, but alternating monthly, Split Dose Method

Thereafter, the patient occasionally would receive a constitutional remedy, and today he continues healthy.

REMARKS

Spongia was selected because of the soft, rubbery consistency of the glands.

CASE 64 [p-P]   *May, 1990*

Male, 43 years, came for homoeopathic treatment because he was starting to experience low-grade fevers—and abnormal glands were appearing in the inguinal, cervical, and supracervical regions.

Biopsy report: Hodgkin's lymphoma, Stage III. CT scan revealed affected mediastinal glands and enlargement of the spleen.

The patient was hot, mildly obese and had a long-standing thyroid condition, for which he never took thyroid substitutes. He was by nature reserved, responsible, and took life seriously. Otherwise, no clear homoeopathic symptoms.

PRESCRIPTION

Months 1-3:   *Aurum iodatum* 200c - weekly, Split Dose Method
Also during this time, whenever the fever rose, the patient took *Pyrogenium* 200c (as needed) and *Arsenicum iodatum* 6x several times a day; this combination would bring down the fever.

During this time, the condition came under control. The cervical and supraclavicular glands vanished and the patient was almost afebrile.

CT scan showed disappearance of mediastinal glands and spleen normal. The only residual symptoms were three inguinal lymph nodes.

Months 4-6:   Same as Months 1-3
The patient was entirely afebrile.

Tests showed no change from previous one.

For three years, patient took occasional doses of *Aurum iodatum*, working up from the 200C to the 10M potency; then *Iodum* 6X, two times a day, was taken for five years longer. He continues to be symptom free and works full-time.

Yearly scans show everything normal, but the three small inguinal glands still persist.

REMARKS

The reasoning behind the selection of the principal remedy is somewhat intricate. *Aurum iodatum*, like some other metal remedies *(Aurum metallicum, Plumbum metallicum, Selenium)* has proven effective for various forms of swollen lymph glands and nodes (adenitis). The fact that the patient felt hot and that the iodine component is extremely useful for thyroid (hence the subsequent *Iodum* 6X prescription) prompted the selection of *Aurum iodatum* rather than the more traditional remedy for Hodgkin's, *Aurum metallicum*.

CASE 65   *March, 1995*

Male, 33 years, presented with a recurrence of Hodgkin's lymphoma. The glands on his neck were soft and rubbery.

> *History: About one year earlier, the patient had started having mild fever almost every day. After a month he visited his doctor, who discovered an abnormal gland in the right supraclavicular region, one in the right armpit, and one in the left inguinal region. An excision biopsy and histopathological report revealed Hodgkin's lymphoma, Stage II. The patient was put on intensive chemotherapy for six months, then on a long-term maintenance dose. Within three months, two more glands appeared on the left side of the cheek—at which point he turned to homoeopathy.*

The patient had a history of tuberculosis diagnosed when he was age 22. It was treated conventionally and cured. He was also prone to skin lesions from time to time, like eczema and contact dermatitis—all of which fit the picture of *Scrophularia nodosa*.

PRESCRIPTION

Week 1:   *Scrophularia nodosa* 200c† - daily, Plussing Method

Week 2:   *Carcinosin* 200c - daily, Plussing Method

Weeks 3-12:   Same as Weeks 1-2
               The glands had resumed normal size. The patient put on weight and felt absolutely normal.

               The chemotherapy was discontinued.

Months 4-6:   Same as Weeks 1-2, but in the 1M potency

               Routine visits to the oncologist showed the blood picture normal. The patient refused the advised maintenance dose of chemotherapy.

For one year thereafter, the patient received single doses of *Scrophularia* 1M and *Carcinosin* 1M, alternating monthly, Split Dose Method; then no more medicines. Almost six years later he is still doing well.

REMARKS

Scrophularia nodosa is "a powerful medicine whenever enlarged glands are present; for Hodgkin's disease" (Boericke). The remedy is especially fitting when there is a patient or family history of tuberculosis in the picture and when, as with *Spongia,* the glands are soft and rubbery.

Dr. Ramakrishnan's Results with Hodgkin's

	No. of Cases	No. of Viable Cases	No. of Successes	Success Rate
Pre-Plussing (<1993)	65	30	15	50%
Plussing (≥1993)	85	47	36	77%

Melanoma

The principal remedies for melanomas, listed in order of frequency of use, are: *Arsenicum album, Arsenicum bromatum, Causticum,* and *Calcarea arsenica.*

CASE 66   *June, 1995*

Female, 28 years, presented with a melanomous lesion on right eyebrow, diagnosed as Stage III.

> *History: The patient had had four melanomas on the face excised during the past two years—all on the right side. CT scan guided biopsy revealed a malignant spot on the liver.*

The woman had a history of a weak bladder: whenever she coughed, sneezed, or laughed suddenly, urine would spurt out. She also mentioned another highly *Causticum* symptom: her spirits would lift and she always felt physically better when it rained; long spells of dry, clear weather would enervate her.

PRESCRIPTION

Week 1:   *Causticum* 200c† - daily, Plussing Method

Week 2:   *Carcinosin* 200c - daily, Plussing Method

Weeks 3-8:   Same as Weeks 1-2
               Lesion completely disappeared.

Months 3-4:   Same as Weeks 1-2

Months 5-8:   Same as Weeks 1-2, but in the 1M potency

Months 9-14:   *Causticum* 1M and *Carcinosin* 1M - alternating semimonthly, Split Dose Method.

> *CT scan showed that the spot on the liver had completely cleared.*

For the next year, the woman received the two remedies in the 10M potency, alternating monthly, Split Dose Method. Then the intensive treatment ended.

> *CT scan was performed every six months for two years. After that, and to date, once a year. All tests show normal.*

REMARKS

Causticum was prescribed both because of the constitutional type and the remedy's affinity with melanomas.

CASE 67   *December, 1994*

Female, 35 years, reported with fast-appearing lesions on face, hand, legs—six areas altogether; all had manifested within the last three months. She experienced intense burning, which lessened after warm applications.

> *Biopsy report: malignant melanoma, Stage III.*

The woman was immaculately dressed, was neat and well organized in her life habits, and she felt better from warmth in every form.

PRESCRIPTION

Week 1:	*Arsenicum album* 200c[†] - daily, Plussing Method
Week 2:	*Carcinosin* 200c - daily, Plussing Method
Weeks 3-16:	Same as Weeks 1-2 The skin improved substantially.
	Routine investigation, however, revealed secondary deposits in the liver and bones.
Week 17:	*Hekla lava* 200c - daily, Plussing Method

Week 18:   *Scirrhinum* 200c - daily, Plussing Method
                  The two remedies were introduced because of this
                  new development.

Weeks 19-28:   Same as Weeks 17-18

                  Testing showed a great reduction of spots.

Months 8-9:   Same as Weeks 17-18

                  *CT scan came out clean with regard to liver and
                  bones.*

Months 10-14: Same as Weeks 1-2, but in the 1M potency.

                  Tests showed everything perfectly normal.

For one year longer, *Arsenicum album* 1M and *Carcinosin* 1M were
alternated monthly, Split Dose Method.

REMARKS

The patient's constitutional picture and modalities promoted the
selection of *Arsenicum album* in both opening and, later, complet-
ing the case.

Carcinosin, rather than *Scirrhinum,* is the preferred nosode for
melanomas. *Scirrhinum* was interpolated specifically to combat
the secondary lesions in the liver. That accomplished, the doctor
returned to *Carcinosin.*

DR. RAMAKRISHNAN'S RESULTS WITH MELANOMAS

	No. of Cases	No. of Viable Cases	No. of Successes	Success Rate
Pre-Plussing (<1993)	40	20	12	60%
Plussing (≥1993)	52	21	15	71%

Skin

The principal remedies for skin cancer (whether basal or squamous), listed in order of frequency of use, are *Arsenicum bromatum, Arsenicum album, Sulphur,* and *Euphorbium.*

CASE 68   *November, 1994*

Female, 29 years, presented with a skin cancer on the left forearm, which had been diagnosed two years previously as squamous cell carcinoma, Stage II. Symptoms were pain and burning. She also had an enlarged left axillary lymph node.

> *History: The woman lived in the South of France, where she spent much time sunbathing. Various allopathic treatments had not helped.*

PRESCRIPTION

Week 1:	*Arsenicum bromatum* 200C - daily, Plussing Method
Week 2:	*Carcinosin* 200C - daily, Plussing Method
Weeks 3-8:	Same as Weeks 1-2 Pain and burning decreased; less serous discharge.
Months 3-4:	Same as Weeks 1-2 Lesion looked much better, as if drying up.
Months 5-8:	Same as Weeks 1-2, but in the 1M potency At end of 32 weeks, the condition had completely cleared up. Also, the left axillary lymph node was no longer palpable.
Months 9-10:	Same as Months 5-8, but alternating monthly, Split Dose Method

Everything continued clear, so no further treatment.

REMARKS

For the selection of *Arsenicum bromatum,* see Chapter 2.

CASE 69   *May, 1996*

Female, 33 years, presented with a badly neglected 8 cm. lesion on the right thigh; it was crater-like, with everted margins and an indurated, sloughing-off base. The whole was infected with a strong odor. The modalities were burning, better from cold applications.

Biopsy diagnosis: Basal cell carcinoma, Stage II.

PRESCRIPTION

Week 1:   *Euphorbium* 200c - daily, Plussing Method

Week 2:   *Carcinosin* 200c - daily, Plussing Method

Weeks 3-8:   Same as Weeks 1-2
               The patient was responding well. The base was clearing up; less infection, less burning.

Months 3-4:   Same as Weeks 1-2
               Slight progress only.

Months 5-8:   Same as Weeks 1-2, but in the 1M potency
               Whole lesion cleared up completely.

No further treatment—and no sign of any ulcer to date.

REMARKS

For the selection of *Euphorbium,* see Chapter 6.

CASE 70   *December, 1995*

Female, 28 years, presented with a 5 cm. lesion on the left thigh that had been neglected for almost a year and was now in a fairly advanced stage. It had a hard, indurated base with sloughing material, everted margins; it bled on touch and was foul smelling.

Biopsy report: Basal cell carcinoma.

The woman came from a small village in the mountains of Northern India. She was an agricultural laborer, uneducated even in the rudiments of good hygiene.

PRESCRIPTION

Week 1:	*Sulphur* 200C - daily, Plussing Method
Week 2:	*Carcinosin* 200C - daily, Plussing Method Additionally. the patient was given *Arsenicum iodatum* 6X, to be taken twice a day. The patient showed substantial progress.
Weeks 3-16:	Same as Weeks 1-2 The patient continued to show rapid progress; the ulcer healed more than 50%.
Months 5-6:	Same as Weeks 1-2, but in the 1M potency The skin lesion healed completely without any residue. *No test or biopsy required because of the complete healing of the skin.*

End of treatment.

REMARKS

Sulphur was selected because of the picture of poor hygiene, foul smell, and because it is preeminent for skin affections in general, including cancers of the skin.

Dr. Ramakrishnan's Results with Skin Cancer

	No. of Cases	No. of Viable Cases*	No. of Successes	Success Rate
Pre-Plussing (<1993)	70	32	18	56%
Plussing (≥1993)	45	35	28	80%

*The viable cases were those that had not already metastasized. Barring a few exceptions, all of the skin cancer cases treated by Dr. Ramakrishnan have been in Southeast Asia, where patients reported only at the middle or later stages of the disease.

Chapter 5
Assistance and Palliation in Cancer Cases That Lie Beyond Homoeopathic Healing

Every homoeopath treating patients who have cancer encounters a large number of cases which, because the malignancy is discovered (or patients come to homoeopathy) only after metastasis has set in, lie beyond the healing powers of the homoeopathic medicines. For example, cancers of the liver and lungs are generally found to be secondary tumors or sites, and therefore later stages of cancer; and uterine, stomach, and pancreatic cancers are usually discovered only when too advanced for cure. Also, a number of leukemia cases fall into this category.

This does not mean, however, that homoeopathy has nothing to offer in the way of palliation and assistance. As will be seen in the cases cited in this chapter, the remedies can significantly relieve pain and discomfort, strengthen the physical condition, improve the mental and emotional state—and generally enhance the quality of a patient's life.

The case examples in this chapter also illustrate the general procedure of employing the Plussing Method for as long as it is effective. (It is extremely important to continue with the method even if the patient is hospitalized and is undergoing allopathic treatment.) After that, in administering the remedies, one follows the procedure described in Chapter 6.

It should be noted that with those patients treated prior to 1993, Dr. Ramakrishnan would today employ the Plussing Method and the more frequent and consistent use of the cancer nosodes to improve their chances of recovery or increase their longevity.

Vocal Cord

CASE 71   *March, 1995*

Male, 53 years, reported with severe hoarseness, pain while talking, enlarged left cervical glands and difficulty in swallowing: diagnosed squamous cell carcinoma of the vocal cord, Stage IV.

> *History: Vocal cord papilloma growth had been*
> *operated on, but twice recurred. Recently, malig-*
> *nant deposits spotted in pharynx, epiglottis, and*
> *also near the uvula. The patient turned to*
> *homoeopathy.*

The patient was a *Lachesis:* of a jealous, suspicious nature, very irritable, and all his symptoms were worse in the morning, especially on waking.

PRESCRIPTION

Week 1:   *Lachesis* 200c† - daily, Plussing Method

Week 2:   *Carcinosin* 200c - daily, Plussing Method

Weeks 3-4:   Same as Weeks 1-2
               The patient felt better, could speak a few words
               without pain, and could swallow easier.

Weeks 5-8:   Same as Weeks 1-2
               The patient continued to feel better overall.

Months 3-4:   Same as Weeks 1-2
               The patient maintained progress.

Months 5-8:   Same as Weeks 1-2, but in the 1M potency
               Spread of disease was restricted during this time.
               When there were episodes of bleeding from nose
               and bloodstained expectoration, additional doses
               of *Lachesis* 1M or *Carcinosin* 1M controlled the
               bleeding.

After eight months of relative comfort and control of the disease, the patient died.

REMARKS

Lachesis not only fit the patient's constitutional picture, but also it is an important remedy for various cancerous throat symptoms and for hemorrhaging.

Oesophagus

CASE 72   *February, 1994*

Male, 64 years, presented with a total obstruction of the oesophagus. He was only able to take small sips of water.

> *Endoscopy showed an obstruction in the middle third of oesophagus where it hit the mass. A biopsy showed a squamous cell carcinoma, Stage IV.*

The patient was a typical *Phosphorus:* of slender build, with small, regular features; a sensitive, amiable disposition; fond of salty foods, ice-cold water, and ice cream.

PRESCRIPTION

Week 1:   *Phosphorus* 200c† - daily, Plussing Method

Week 2:   *Carcinosin* 200c - daily, Plussing Method
               A steady progress was discernible.

Weeks 3-4:   Same as Weeks 1-2
               Progress continued to the point at which patient could take semisoft food, such as porridge with milk, puréed vegetables, etc.

Months 2-3:   Same as Weeks 1-2

Months 4-6:   Same as Weeks 1-2, but in the 1M potency
               The patient was completely comfortable and could eat semisolid food.

Months 7-9:   Same as Weeks 1-2, but in the 10M potency
               The patient continued free of pain and enjoying life.

During the tenth month, there was a sudden spasm from total obstruction. The patient could not even drink water without vomiting bright red blood. At this point, he quickly slipped into labored breathing and died.

Breast

CASE 73 *June, 1995*

Female, 43 years, presented with a cancer of the right breast, Stage IV. The primary lesion was an open wound, with a hard, indurated base, everted margins, and a foul discharge. The patient was experiencing burning pains in many parts of her body (where the cancer had metastasized), which were relieved by cold applications.

> *History: In October, 1993, a radical mastectomy of the left breast had been performed, followed by radiation therapy. Early in 1995, there was a recurrence in the right breast, and a combination of radiation therapy and chemotherapy was attempted. This only exacerbated patient's condition, and the cancer metastasized to the lungs, liver, ribs, and skull.*

PRESCRIPTION

Week 1:   *Euphorbium* 200c - daily, Plussing Method

Week 2:   *Sulphur* 200c - daily, Plussing Method
              The patient felt better: pain and burning
              subsided.

Weeks 3-16:   Same as Weeks 1-2
              Excellent response. All pain and burning vanished. The patient ate and slept better, even felt as if she might recover.

Weeks 17-18: Same as Weeks 1-2

During the fifth month, there was a massive hemorrhage from the breast wound (and probably also internally) and, within a few hours, the woman passed away.

REMARKS

Sulphur was prescribed, in part for the foul-smelling discharge, in part for the burning pain.

Euphorbium is a most effective remedy for the palliation stages of cancer—especially when there is severe burning which is relieved by cold applications, even though the patient is usually chilly *(see Chapter 6)*.

No cancer nosode was used, since the case was too advanced, and only palliation of symptoms was being attempted (see Case 77).

Lung

CASE 74 [p-P]   *November, 1988*

Male, 72 years, reported with a diagnosed adenocarcinoma of the lungs, Stage IV. His symptoms were an intractable cough, rapid loss of weight, and physical and mental weakness.

> *Bronchoscopy had shown huge lesions on both lungs, with almost entire lungs destroyed. Lungs were the secondary site. A detailed CT scan and colonoscopy found the primary lesion on the cecum—which was asymptomatic.*

The patient was touchy, angry, unmanageable in his illness—and by nature, arrogant.

PRESCRIPTION

Weeks 1-3:	*Lycopodium* 200c† - weekly, Split Dose Method
Week 4:	*Carcinosin* 200c - weekly, Split Dose Method
Month 2:	Same as Week 1 The patient's condition improved.
Month 3:	*Nitricum acidum* 200c - weekly, Split Dose Method The condition improved further. The cough was under control, the patient gained 6 lb. and was now reasonably comfortable.
Months 4-6:	The patient developed a number of symptoms, including severe distention of the abdomen, relieved by belching, for which he would be prescribed *Carbo vegetabilis* 200c, a dose taken every hour, ten times.

> *CT scan showed no deterioration of his condition.*

Month 7:   *Lycopodium* 200c and *Carbo vegetabilis* 200c - alternating weekly, Split Dose Method

Months 8-10:   Same as Month 7, but in the 1M potency.

Months 11-12:   Same as Month 7, but in the 10M potency.
                The patient was comfortable, his condition stable.

At this point, one year after beginning homoeopathic treatment, the patient developed multiple secondary lesions in the brain and died shortly thereafter.

REMARKS

Lycopodium was prescribed both for its affinity with the lungs and for the personality picture.

Nitricum acidum was prescribed to address the primary tumor in the cecum.

CASE 75 [p-P]   *April, 1991*

Male, 56 years, a heavy smoker for forty years, presented with diagnosed bronchogenic carcinoma, Stage IV. The lesion was right-sided, with the typical *Lycopodium* early-evening aggravation.

> *Tests showed metastasis in the bones, ribs, vertebrae, shoulder, etc.—also in the brain and liver.*

PRESCRIPTION

Week 1:   *Lycopodium* 200c - weekly, Split Dose Method

Week 2:   *Carcinosin* 200c - weekly, Split Dose Method

Weeks 3-16:   Same as Weeks 1-2
              The patient felt comfortable all this time. When there was any bleeding, from the lungs, he would take *Sanguinaria* 200c, ten times at half-hour intervals, and that would arrest the bleeding.

Week 17:   The patient developed shortness of breath and respiratory failure. Ventilator therapy was initiated, and he died in three days.

REMARKS

No other medicines were given during the four months of homoeopathic treatment, except vitamins and a sleeping pill. Until the very end the patient was comfortable, looked cheerful, and even gained a little weight. He took a small vacation during this time, and at other times friends and relatives dropped by to socialize. His death was peaceful.

CASE 76   *January, 1998*

Male, 73 years, presented with a Stage IV huge (baseball size) swelling over the left clavicle, which was stony hard and immovable. He had been a heavy smoker, and the primary cancer was in the lung.

> *History: Lung cancer diagnosed in 1991. The patient underwent surgery, radiation, chemotherapy. But in the last six months, the left supraclavicular gland started swelling up.*

The patient was extremely cold, as well as restless. By nature, he was critical, fastidious, and always teaching others how to live their lives—a typical *Arsenicum album.*

PRESCRIPTION

Week 1:   *Arsenicum album* 200C - daily, Plussing Method

Week 2:   *Scirrhinum* 200C - daily, Plussing Method

Weeks 3-6:   Same as Weeks 1-2
              The patient attested to great relief from symptoms when taking *Arsenicum album,* and much less when taking *Scirrhinum.*

Weeks 7-15:   Same as Weeks 1-2, but switched to *Carcinosin* 200C instead of *Scirrhinum*

The patient made a dramatic temporary recovery during this time. But there was no scope for a true recovery and, during Week 16, he deteriorated swiftly and passed away peacefully.

REMARKS

Two points came out clearly in this case: (1) There was a definite improvement in pain relief when the prescriber switched to *Carcinosin*. Why this was so is unclear, but one must remain open to the possibility that the second cancer nosode may work, if the first does not. (2) *Arsenicum album,* as it so often does, relieved severe pain and major discomfort until the end.

CASE 77   *February, 1993*

Female, 71 years, came for homoeopathic treatment for her diagnosed adenocarcinoma of the lungs, with positive malignant deposits in lymph nodes, Stage IV. She was coughing and experienced pain in the right pectoral region.

> *History: Primary tumor in the right ovary had been operated on, December, 1989. In January, 1991, secondary lesions were discovered in the right lung, axilla, and supraclavicular region. Chemotherapy and radiation therapy were not tolerated and hence were abandoned.*

The woman had a history of tuberculosis, diagnosed when she was twenty years old, for which she was treated for two years.

PRESCRIPTION

Week 1:   *Lapis albus* 200C - daily, Plussing Method

Week 2:   *Tuberculinum bovinum* 200C - daily, Plussing Method
The patient felt slightly better.

Weeks 3-8:   Same as Weeks 1-2
The patient felt much better. No cough, no pain, gained 2 lb.

Months 3-4:   Same as Weeks 1-2
The axilla and supraclavicular nodes were much smaller.

> *CT scan showed secondary deposits unaltered in size.*

Months 5-6:   Same as Weeks 1-2, but in the 1M potency
The patient continued to do well.

For the two following years, the patient would receive periodic doses of *Lapis albus* 1M or *Tuberculinum bovinum* 1M and continued to do well. After two years the lesion in the lung started growing and the liver and spleen showed signs of deterioration; and the patient died a few months later.

REMARKS

Lapis albus has proven of benefit in cancerous affections of the lungs, especially when there is a tubercular background.

Tuberculinum was chosen because of the history of tuberculosis. Since this remedy stepped in as the nosode—and since, realistically speaking, the objective was palliation rather than cure—no cancer nosode was used (see Case 73).

Stomach

CASE 78   *February, 1994*

Male, 46 years, with a history of stomach cancer, presented with an upper abdominal pain. Symptoms were intense burning in epigastrium, acidity, sudden pain in upper abdomen, and a coffee-colored vomitus.

> *History: Endoscopy had revealed a one-inch diameter ulcer, which was biopsied. Histopathology report: Adenocarcinoma of stomach, Stage IIIb. There were secondary lesions in the liver and in the T10 vertebra. Total gastrectomy was performed, followed by chemotherapy and radiation therapy. Three months later, the patient again developed pain in the abdomen. At this point he turned to homoeopathy.*

PRESCRIPTION

Week 1:   *Hydrastis* 200c - daily, Plussing Method

Week 2:   *Carcinosin* 200c - daily, Plussing Method

Weeks 3-4:   Same as Weeks 1-2
               Excellent relief—patient felt better than he had for the past year.

Weeks 5-16:   Same as Weeks 1-2
               The patient continued to feel well, but by Week 15, water retention was slowly setting in: oedema of feet, ascites, breathlessness.

Week 17:   *Apis* 200c - daily, Plussing Method

Week 18:   *Carcinosin* 200c - daily, Plussing Method
               The patient passed large quantities of urine; retention was significantly less, but now there was burning in the abdomen, ameliorated by cold applications—for which *Euphorbium* 30c was prescribed, one dose every hour, ten times.

Weeks 19-22:   *Hydrastis* 1M and *Carcinosin* 1M - alternating
daily, Plussing Method
The patient felt fairly comfortable during this
time.

By Week 23, there was a huge metastasis in the lungs, pleural effusion, and the patient died.

REMARKS

In sum, the patient lived for almost six months after beginning homoeopathy—during which time he felt well. The end was swift and peaceful.

Apis was prescribed for the picture that emerged in Week 15. As was seen already in Case 60, it is an excellent remedy for oedematous conditions (see also Case 86).

For the selection of *Euphorbium,* see Chapter 6.

CASE 79   *January, 1995*

Male, 66 years, presented after a stomach cancer operation and the removal of 23 of 30 mesenteric glands—all malignant; Stage IV.

> *Surgical procedures and tests showed that the*
> *cancer had metastasized to the liver, spleen, and*
> *pancreas.*

The patient's constitutional picture pointed to *Argentum nitricum*. He displayed a fear of heights and flying and an anxiety for all simple, everyday events. He also suffered from hand tremors, periodic right-sided nosebleeds, and was mildly diabetic.

PRESCRIPTION

Week 1:   *Argentum nitricum* 200C[†] - daily, Plussing Method

Week 2:   *Carcinosin* 200C - daily, Plussing Method

Weeks 3-4:   Same as Weeks 1-2
                 The patient felt better, could eat better; gained
                 3 lb.

Weeks 5-8:   Same as Weeks 1-2
                 The patient continued to feel better and gained an
                 additional pound.

Weeks 9-16:   Same as Weeks 1-2
                 The patient continued comfortable and stable.

At the end of Week 16, patient developed jaundice.

> *Total serum bilirubin 6 mg./dL.; SGOT 83; SGPT*
> *123.*

Week 17:   *Chelidonium* 200C - daily, Plussing Method

Week 18:   *Scirrhinum* 200C - daily, Plussing Method

> *Total serum bilirubin dropped to 2.5 mg./dL.;*
> *SGOT 56; SGPT 98.*

Weeks 19-35:   Same as Weeks 17-18

> *Blood tests showed that bilirubin and transami-*
> *nases had remained at the same level. The second-*
> *ary lesions in the liver had not increased.*

Week 36:   *Argentum nitricum* 1M - daily, Plussing Method

Week 37:   *Scirrhinum* 1M - daily, Plussing Method

Weeks 38-43:   Same as Weeks 36-37
                 The patient was comfortable all this time.

Week 44:   Sudden severe ascites brought on a coma, and the
                 patient died within a week without regaining con-
                 sciousness.

Summary: The patient lived comfortably and in good spirits for
ten months—even though the cancer was in Stage IV, with metas-
tases in the liver, pancreas, and other organs and in glands all over
the body.

REMARKS

Treatment was switched to *Scirrhinum* in Week 18, when the liver symptoms became more prominent, because usually cancer of the liver responds to this nosode better than to *Carcinosin*.

The use of *Chelidonium* was dictated by the patient's jaundice and the remedy's effectiveness in liver cancer *(see Chapter 2)*.

CASE 80   *January, 1995*

Male, 37 years, presented with the complaint of continuous vomiting—blackish, foul-smelling matter. He was extremely weak and emaciated.

> *History: Six months previously, the patient had been operated on for stomach cancer, diagnosed as adenocarcinoma, Stage IV. The surgery was extensive. The stomach, duodenum, nine inches of small intestine and three-quarters of the pancreas, also the spleen and omentum were removed, as were thirty-two glands. Surgery was followed with chemotherapy.*

PRESCRIPTION

Week 1:   *Cadmium sulphuratum* 200c - daily, Plussing Method

Week 2:   *Carcinosin* 200c - daily, Plussing Method
              Vomiting stopped completely during this time.

Weeks 3-4:   Same as Weeks 1-2
              The patient was comfortable, but still weak.

Month 2:   Same as Weeks 1-2
              No pain at all. Abdomen felt soft and normal. The patient could eat sparingly at short intervals; 1 lb. weight gain.

Blood tests showed that the tumor marker was rising. The attending oncologist wished to start a new chemotherapy drug. The patient refused, choosing to continue with homoeopathy.

Month 3:   Same as Weeks 1-2
             The patient continued to feel slightly better. Condition stable.

Month 4:   The patient complained of burning in abdomen and was switched to *Arsenicum album* 200c, alternating weekly with *Carcinosin* 200c - daily, Plussing Method
             Little difference in symptoms.

Months 5-8: *Cadmium sulphuratum* 1M - daily, Plussing Method
             The patient was much more comfortable.

During Month 9, the patient began vomiting blackish material again and died within a week.

REMARKS

Cadmium sulphuratum (see Chapters 2 and 6) kept the patient reasonably comfortable and well during the eight months that he was taking the remedy.

Pancreas

CASE 81 [p-P]   *June, 1988*

Male, 65 years, presented with a case of pancreatic cancer with secondary deposits in the liver, Stage IV.

> *History: Surgery had removed two-thirds of the cancerous mass at the head of the pancreas, also twenty-eight mesenteric glands, all of them positive; followed by chemotherapy. No other form of treatment was suggested, and the patient turned to homoeopathy.*

The patient had a lot of flatulence, with distention of the abdomen. He was also air-hungry and wanted a fan blowing on his face—a typical *Carbo vegetabilis* picture.

PRESCRIPTION

Week 1:   *Carbo vegetabilis* 200c† - weekly, Split Dose Method

Week 2:   *Carcinosin* 200c - weekly, Split Dose Method

Weeks 3-4:   Same as Weeks 1-2

> *Serum bilirubin came down from 7 to 4.5 mg./dL., alkaline phosphates from 1183 to 905.*

Months 2-4:   Same as Weeks 1-2
               The patient felt much better.

Months 5-8:   Same as Weeks 1-2, but in the 1M potency
               The patient was active, energetic, drove his car, and felt healthy.

> *Serum bilirubin 2.5 mg./dL.; alkaline phosphatase 327.*

In the ninth month, the patient began to lose ground and died within the next two months. During this time, *Chelidonium* and *Natrum sulphuricum* were given for relief of liver pain and discomfort; also *Ceanothus americanus*. These remedies were prescribed on an as needed basis, and interchanged as the symptoms indicated *(see Chapter 6)*.

Liver

CASE 82   *August, 1995*

Male, 53 years, presented with an enlarged liver and spleen and loss of appetite.

> *CT scan and biopsy revealed that squamous cell carcinoma in the liver was secondary, Stage IIIb. The primary site could not be detected.*

PRESCRIPTION

Week 1:	*Chelidonium* 200c - daily, Plussing Method
Week 2:	*Scirrhinum* 200c - daily, Plussing Method
Weeks 3-4:	Same as Weeks 1-2 Slight return of appetite. Perhaps 10% improvement.
Month 2:	Same as Weeks 1-2 Another slight improvement in appetite, and the patient gained 1 lb.
Months 3-6:	Same as Weeks 1-2, but in the 1M potency Slight improvement continued all around. The patient was comfortable.
Months 7-9:	Same as Month 3 The patient continued stable and comfortable.

During Week 38, the patient developed ascites and pulmonary oedema and died quietly.

REMARKS

Here again, one encounters the effectiveness of the organ-specific remedy *Chelidonium* and the cancer nosode *Scirrhinum* in cancers of the liver.

CASE 83   *May, 1993*

Female, 62 years, presented with secondary deposits in the liver and in a number of mesenteric glands.

> *A CT scan–guided biopsy revealed Stage IV adeno-carcinoma. No surgery was performed because no primary site was discovered.*

The woman was a diabetic and had had several bouts of malaria. Both conditions had, in the past, responded well to *Natrum sulphuricum.*

PRESCRIPTION

Week 1:	*Chelidonium* 200c - daily, Plussing Method
Week 2:	*Natrum sulphuricum* 200c† - daily, Plussing Method
Weeks 3-8:	Same as Weeks 1-2 The patient was comfortable.
Months 3-4:	Same as Weeks 1-2, but in the 1M potency The patient did better every week.
Months 5-8:	Same as Months 3-4 The patient felt extremely well.
Month 9:	*Chelidonium* 10M - semimonthly, Split Dose Method
Month 10:	*Natrum sulphuricum* 10M - semimonthly, Split Dose Method The patient continued to feel extremely well.

For two more years, the woman periodically received *Natrum sulphuricum* or *Chelidonium,* in the 10M potency, Split Dose Method—as her symptoms dictated. Then there was an intestinal hemorrhage and the woman died within two weeks.

REMARKS

Chelidonium, as an organ specific remedy, and *Natrum sulphuricum,* as a fitting constitutional remedy, were so effective (given Stage IV, with secondaries in the liver) that Dr. Ramakrishnan judged it best not to change the prescription, and no cancer nosode was employed. To repeat, when the objective is palliation and not cure, the cancer nosode is sometimes omitted (see also Cases 73 and 77).

Colon

CASE 84   *September, 1994*

Male, 52 years, presented with a recurrence of an adenocarcinoma of the colon, Stage IV. The patient had severe pain in the abdomen, which was not relieved by any of the usual analgesics. Pain was due partly to adhesions, and the liver was hard and tender.

History: In July, 1993, a hemicolectomy was performed, followed by chemotherapy. In June, 1994, there was a recurrence in his descending colon with involvement of the liver and nodes in the posterior abdominal wall. A few rounds of chemotherapy were tried, but these did not relieve the patient's discomfort.

PRESCRIPTION

Week 1:   *Graphites* 200c - daily, Plussing Method

Week 2:   *Scirrhinum* 200c - daily, Plussing Method

Weeks 3-4: Same as Weeks 1-2
            Excellent pain relief.

Months 2-4: Same as Weeks 1-2
            Condition stable. The patient put on some weight. Went back to work.

Months 5-8: Same as Weeks 1-2, but in the 1M potency
            Liver became smaller and no pain at all. The patient continued going to work.

            At about nine months, the patient's condition began to deteriorate. The liver grew larger and more tender, there was fluid in the abdomen, and deposits appeared in spleen and lungs.

Months 9-12: *Lycopodium* 200c and *Scirrhinum* 1M, alternating weekly - daily, Plussing Method

With these remedies the patient held his ground. He was comfortable and could work part-time.

Then, at the end of the twelfth month, the condition deteriorated further and the patient died soon after.

REMARKS

For the *Graphites* prescription, see comments on adhesions on pp. 198-199.

Lycopodium was introduced because of lung and liver symptoms.

Ovary

CASE 85 [p-P]   *September, 1990*

Female, 40 years, presented with a metastasized ovarian cancer, Stage IV. She was suffering from acute colicky pains, had fluid in the abdomen, and could hardly eat.

> *History: A large right-sided ovarian adenocarcinoma had been diagnosed adhering to the uterine wall. There was also a lump detected on the left ovary and there was malignancy in several mesenteric glands. The patient was treated with chemotherapy for six months, but the response was not good and she was told that she had only three to four weeks to live. At this point she turned to homoeopathy.*

The woman had a long history of dysmenorrhea.

PRESCRIPTION

Days 1-4:   *Viburnum prunifolium* 200c - to be mixed in a glass of water and sipped every five minutes until she felt better. This procedure, which she repeated frequently, gave her substantial physical relief and she felt more cheerful.

Days 5-15:   *Carcinosin* 200c - once, Split Dose Method, followed by *Viburnum prunifolium* 200c, as needed, for 10 days
The patient was free from pain. The accumulation of fluid in the abdomen had reduced considerably and the patient could eat better. Also, now she was strong enough to go to the toilet by herself (which she could not do previously).

Week 3:   *Viburnum prunifolium* 200c - daily, Split Dose Method

Week 4:   *Carcinosin* 200c - daily, Split Dose Method

Months 2-3:   Same as Weeks 3-4
The patient continued comfortable until the fourth month, when there was profuse vaginal bleeding, which could not be controlled by either homoeopathy or conventional drugs—and the patient passed away swiftly.

REMARKS

See Remarks in Case 6.

CASE 86 [p-P]   *October, 1990*

Female, 37 years, presented with a recurrence of adenocarcinoma on the right ovary, Stage IV. Her symptoms were discomfort from a large accumulation of fluid in the abdomen and despite a general thirstlessness, a craving for milk.

> *History: In January, 1989, surgery had been attempted; the diagnosed ovarian adenocarcinoma could not be fully removed. Surgery was followed by chemotherapy, and the condition was stable for more than one year. A recurrence on the same and also the left side and ascites prompted the patient to seek homoeopathic assistance.*

PRESCRIPTION

Week 1:   *Apis* 200c - once, Split Dose Method
Ascites came down by 2 inches (from 45 to 43 inches). The patient felt better and hopeful.

Week 2:   *Carcinosin* 200c - once, Split Dose Method

Weeks 3-6:   Same as Weeks 1-2
The patient continued to feel better. Abdominal girth down by 6 inches.

During this time, she complained once of severe neuralgic pain from the abdomen radiating down the thighs. *Arsenicum album,* taken on an as-needed basis, helped.

Weeks 7-12:   Same as Weeks 1-2
The patient continued to improve. Cancer appeared to be controlled.

Months 4-6:   *Apis* 200c and *Carcinosin* 200c - alternating semimonthly
The patient continued to feel comfortable.

At the end of six months, the tumor started growing again. The abdomen grew larger. Severe pain was controlled by *Aconite,* when the shooting pains became unbearable and the patient could not lie still one moment; by *Arsenicum album,* when the patient, who was usually stoical, would begin incessantly to complain and find fault with everything around her, and the pain would drive her out of bed to pace the room; and by *Magnesia phosphorica,* when the patient wanted to lie in the fetal position with a heating pad pressed against the painful area. All were prescribed on an as-needed basis, switching from one to the other when one ceased to work (see Case 93). The woman died during her seventh month of homoeopathic treatment.

REMARKS

Apis, as was noted earlier, is a remedy to be considered when there is ascites or much fluid and swelling in the area affected (see Cases 60 and 78), especially when accompanied by thirstlessness.

Uterus

CASE 87 [p-P]   *March, 1989*

Female, 43 years, presented with an advanced uterine cancer. Her symptoms were constant pain in the lower abdomen and profuse, fifteen-day menstrual periods with much clotting.

> *History: During a D&C, a uterine mass 6 cm. ×*
> *5 cm. was detected; the histopathological report*
> *showed adenocarcinoma, Stage IVb. The cancer*
> *had metastasized and the surrounding area was*
> *full of small lumps; there were also deposits in the*
> *liver, lungs, and mesenteric glands. The patient re-*
> *fused to have surgery and turned to homoeopathy.*

The woman was heat intolerant and also intolerant of any tight clothes around her neck, torso, or thighs. She was vivacious, strong-minded, and admitted to jealousy—a perfect picture of *Lachesis.*

PRESCRIPTION

Weeks 1-2:   *Lachesis* 200c† - weekly, Split Dose Method

Weeks 3-4:   Same as Week 1
               Some improvement.

Month 2:   Same as Week 1
               The patient definitely better. Less pain.

               Mass was the same in size. No changes seen.

Months 3-10:   *Lachesis* 200c and *Aurum muriaticum natronatum* 200c - alternating weekly, Split Dose Method
               Case held well and patient felt comfortable.

Month 11:   The patient developed ascites and no longer re- sponded to any remedies. A profuse hemorrhage occurred; the patient was hospitalized and died shortly thereafter.

CASE 88 [p-P]   *January, 1988*

Female, 58 years, presented with a diagnosed uterine cancer. She was experiencing pain, weakness, and great sadness.

> *CT scan followed by a D&C confirmed adenocarcinoma of the uterus, Stage IIIb. The patient refused all treatment except homoeopathy.*

The woman was of a sympathetic nature, sensitive and considerate of others. She preferred salt to sweet and, eight years previously, had had a papilloma of the vocal cord removed—all of which suggested *Causticum*.

PRESCRIPTION

Weeks 1-2:   *Causticum* 200c† - weekly, Split Dose Method

Week 3-6:   Same as Week 1
                Some slight improvement.

> *CT scan indicated no change.*

Weeks 7-12:   Same as Week 1, but in the 1M potency
                For the first time, patient had no pain, was less weak, cheerful, and had gained a few pounds.

Month 4:   *Aurum muriaticum natronatum* 200c - weekly, Split Dose Method
                The patient continued to improve, was now comfortable and asymptomatic.

For the next three years, until August, 1991, *Causticum* 1M and *Aurum muriaticum natronatum* 1M, alternating monthly, Split Dose Method, kept the woman in a stable condition, comfortable and asymptomatic. But in September, 1991, the cancer started to metastasize to the abdomen, lungs, and axillary glands—and the patient died a couple of months later.

REMARKS

Once again, the effectiveness of *Aurum muriaticum natronatum*, as an organ specific remedy for cancers of the female reproductive system, is observed *(see Chapters 2 and 9)*.

CASE 89 [p-P]   *June, 1986*

Female, 41 years, presented with a painful, swollen abdomen (she looked about 20 weeks pregnant), profuse leucorrhea, emaciation, and shortness of breath, even at rest. There was significant weight loss.

> *Tests diagnosed adenocarcinoma of the uterus, with secondaries in liver, lungs, mesenteric glands; Stage IV.*

The patient was a typical *Arsenicum album:* extremely sensitive to cold, restless, fastidious, fault-finding, and constantly complaining; pain not relieved in any position, but some relief from a hot water bottle.

PRESCRIPTION

Week 1:	*Arsenicum album* 200c† - daily, Split Dose Method. Pain was significantly decreased and the patient looked more cheerful.
Week 2:	Same as Week 1. Pain was almost gone. The patient had more energy and complained less.
Weeks 3-6:	Same as Week 1, but weekly. The patient continued to look better—although weight remained the same.
Weeks 7-12:	Carcinosin 200c - weekly, Split Dose Method. The patient's condition remained stable. No pain and very little discomfort, although the slightest exertion made her breathless.

Months 4-6:   *Arsenicum album* 1M and *Carcinosin* 1M - alternating semimonthly, Split Dose Method

Although she spent most of her time in bed, the woman was comfortable and read a great deal of the time. These six months under homoeopathic treatment were the most peaceful and pain-free months of the entire two-year span of her sickness. In December, the patient developed jaundice, with high bilirubin and liver enzymes, and died shortly thereafter.

Bone

CASE 90   *September, 1993*

Female, 56 years, presented with secondary cancer lesions in the fourth lumbar vertebrae, Stage IV.

> *History: In June, 1993, patient was diagnosed with poorly differentiated cell carcinoma in the right kidney. Radical nephrectomy immediately performed. September, 1993, a routine scan detected secondary lesions in the L4 region. Radiation therapy was advised, but the patient refused and turned to homoeopathy.*

The woman was a typical *Natrum muriaticum:* suffering from frequent headaches and depression since childhood; worse from the sun and humidity; constipated and craving salt. She also had a history of broken or unsatisfactory relationships with family and friends.

PRESCRIPTION

Week 1:   *Hekla lava* 200c - daily, Plussing Method

Week 2:   *Carcinosin* 200c- daily, Plussing Method

Weeks 3-8:   Same as Weeks 1-2
             Lesions were completely gone.

Months 3-6: Same as Weeks 1-2

End of intensive treatment.

For three years, the patient did well on *Natrum muriaticum* 1M† and *Carcinosin* 1M, alternating monthly, Split Dose Method. Then she developed ascites due to multiple lesions in her mesenteric glands and died within a couple of months.

REMARKS

Today Dr. Ramakrishnan would have continued the Plussing Method longer—which might have increased the woman's longevity.

Leukemia

CASE 91   *June, 1997*

Male, 54 years, presented with a case of diagnosed myelodysplas-tic syndrome or myelogenous leukemia, Stage IV.

> *History: The patient first went to the doctor for an unremitting fever that was not responding to any drug. His total white blood count (WBC) was 2500, and the differential showed myelocytes and metamyelocytes, which persisted throughout his illness. Bone marrow smear and biopsy revealed features of myelodysplastic syndrome with excess blasts. Chemotherapy for the present and a bone marrow transplant for the future were advised. The patient refused all forms of conventional treatment and turned to homoeopathy.*

The patient suffered from extreme weakness, some shortness of breath, recurrent fevers—and looked extremely pale.

PRESCRIPTION

Week 1:   *Hekla lava* 200c - daily, Plussing Method

Week 2:   *Carcinosin* 200c - daily, Plussing Method

Weeks 3-8:   Same as Weeks 1-2
               The patient felt fairly comfortable, febrile episodes less severe.

               > *The blood cell count (CBC), monitored regularly, revealed no deterioration of the condition.*

Weeks 9-16:   Same as Weeks 1-2
               The patient looked less anemic. Two episodes of bleeding gums during this time were controlled with *Phosphorus* 200c - one dose every hour, ten times.

> *Tests showed the leukopenia improved; total count had risen to 3700. But there was extreme shortness of breath and some fluid in the base of the lungs.*

Week 17:   *Lycopodium* 200c - daily, Plussing Method

Week 18:   *Carcinosin* 200c - daily, Plussing Method
               The patient felt better.

Weeks 19-24:   Same as Weeks 17-18
               The patient continued to feel comfortable.

In the seventh month, the patient developed a massive infection of the liver. Several homoeopathic remedies were tried *(Arsenicum album, Chelidonium, Phosphorus, Natrum sulphuricum),* in addition to antibiotics—but to no avail. The patient died shortly thereafter.

REMARKS

Lycopodium was selected because of the increasing lung symptoms.

CASE 92 [p-P]   *September, 1992*

Female, 26 years, presented with diagnosed non-Hodgkin's leukemia, Stage IV. She had multiple malignant glands all over the body: cervical, axilla, inguinal, mediastinal, abdominal—and daily fevers.

> *Blood tests: High percentage of immature cells, hemoglobin 4.3 gm./dL. Various chemotherapeutic drugs were tried, but were ineffective in the case. When these efforts were exhausted, the patient turned to homoeopathy.*

The woman had a history of respiratory illnesses, which would start with a sore throat, then proceed to and lodge in the lungs. She also had had a couple of bouts of pneumonia.

PRESCRIPTION

Week 1:   *Phosphorus* 200c† - once, Split Dose Method
               Also, *Arsenicum album* 30c for fever - 10 doses on
               an hourly basis (when needed)
               The patient felt slightly better.

Weeks 2-3:   Same as Week 1
               The patient was free of fever. She looked better,
               had more energy.

               Hemoglobin report: 4.8 gm./dL.

Week 4:   *Carcinosin* 200c - once, Split Dose Method

Month 2:   Same as Week 1
               Relief continued. The patient was cheerful,
               afebrile, and looked less toxic.

               Hemoglobin level slowly rising.

In the ninth week, the patient suddenly developed jaundice, went
into a coma, and passed away quietly within two days.

REMARKS

Phosphorus was selected because of the woman's respiratory tract
history.

Arsenicum album has proven to be extremely valuable in reducing
fevers in leukemia cases.

Chapter 6
Pain Control in the Advanced and Terminal Stages of Cancer

At the present time, and until homoeopathy becomes more widely recognized in the Western world, a large number of cancer patients seek homoeopathic assistance only after they have reached Stage IV or the terminal stage of the disease—when the primary tumors are fixed and pressing on the surrounding areas, and secondary lesions are widespread in the body. But as was observed in Chapter 5, sometimes the remedies will sufficiently strengthen the life force to permit a patient to pursue his former interests and occupations during his (or her) remaining time. At the very least, they should materially alleviate the pain or discomfort. And on rare occasions, the recovery of a seemingly terminal case (such as Case 31) will partake of the nature of a miracle.

There are almost no rules or formulas for the advanced stages of cancer, as the homoeopath finds himself responding to the fluctuations and twists and turns of a patient's condition. But there are some general procedures that one can fall back upon—and, above all, there is a group of pain-relieving remedies that are effective when the cancer nosode, organ-specific, or constitutional remedy are of no avail.

Principal Remedies Used

The most prominent palliative remedies, in alphabetical order, are discussed first.

ACONITE. For shooting pains that come on suddenly and last a long time. Pains accompanied by great physical and mental restlessness. Often symptoms are worse at night and/or in a stuffy room. But pains, especially the neuralgia type, can be alleviated by warmth. At times there will be a fear of death which comes on in the middle of the night—often in the form of a panic attack (see Case 93).

ARSENICUM ALBUM. Probably *the* most often used remedy in cancer palliation. The patient is extremely restless, tosses and turns in bed, is unable to find a comfortable position, and wants to get up and walk about. He moves from bed to sofa and back again, from room to room, or paces the room—not finding relief anywhere. Great exhaustion, weakness, and debility are present. There are burning pains that are relieved by heat. Nightly aggravations (especially between midnight and 4:00 a.m.) occurs. Often there is a constant thirst or dryness of mouth that is not quenched by frequent sips of liquid. A great deal of fear and anxiety and mental restlessness accompanies all complaints. The patient is critical and sensitive to disorder around him, and even when extremely ill, still directs the caretaker what to do. He fears being left alone, fears death, and feels it is useless to take medicines.

AURUM METALLICUM—FOR BONE PAINS. Used in sarcomas, osteomyelitis, secondaries in bones, when pains are intolerable (see Case 58), often worse at night, and the patient is worse from cold, better from warmth—but likes fresh air. The mental picture might be one of severe depression.

CADMIUM SULPHURATUM—ESPECIALLY FOR STOMACH. This remedy is called for when there is much nausea, burning and persistent vomiting (of blackish, coffee-ground matter). A dose administered every half-hour throughout the day (and night) brings the desired relief. The remedy is also a major one for the nausea and vomiting that often accompany or follow chemotherapy *(see Chapter 8)*.

CHELIDONIUM. This remedy was described in Chapter 2. Here one need only add that it is invaluable for the pain of cancers that have metastasized to the liver. It can be used alone for as long as it is effective—or it can be alternated with other remedies, as needed. Usually the 200C potency works best.

EUPHORBIUM. "Pains of cancer" (Boericke). *Burning* pains characterize this remedy (see Cases 73 and 78); the patient does not like cool air *but* feels better with cold applications. The remedy resembles *Arsenicum album* in its restlessness and intensity of pain, but differs from the latter in its amelioration from cold.

HYDRASTIS. This remedy was described in Chapter 2. In the terminal stage, the principal symptoms are prostration, extreme pain, and sometimes obstinate constipation.

MAGNESIA PHOSPHORICA. Pain is due to spasms or cramping of muscles, with radiating pain; the patient wants to bend over double and apply pressure and warmth to painful area to obtain relief (see Case 86). Best method of administration: dissolve a dose of the remedy in the 30th potency in a cup of *warm* water, and take 1 teaspoon every 5 minutes, 10 times. Repeat as necessary, raising the potency as necessary.

NUX VOMICA. The patient is nervous, testy, irritable, hypersensitive to odor, light, noise, etc. He has a low tolerance for pain, may not want to be touched, and is impatient; time passes too slowly. He might also be more than usually fault-finding with his caretaker and of everything and everyone around him. There is much nausea, with or without vomiting; the patient wants to vomit but cannot. The patient's complaints are worse in the morning, from eating; better after a nap, in the evening, and with application of warmth. Apart from affording relief in conditions where the liver is involved and the nausea is severe, *Nux* has been found to be useful when a patient is no longer responding to *Arsenicum album* and needs a rest from that remedy. After giving *Nux* for a while, the patient will once again respond to *Arsenicum* (see Case 93).

OPIUM—NOT AVAILABLE IN THE UNITED STATES, BUT AVAILABLE IN THE UNITED KINGDOM, WESTERN EUROPE, AND INDIA. The potentized opium's modalities are worse from heat and after sleep (patient sleeps into an aggravation, like *Lachesis*); better after cold applications, also from fresh air, small quantities of food, and walking about. *Opium* is used in conditions in which hard glands press on the abdominal organs, peritoneum, or brain. Other symptoms are fluid causing distention; deposits in liver or metastasized to spleen, pancreas, lungs, or mediastinum; pain leading to severe depression.

The remedy also has the capacity to bring a patient out of a coma, especially a hepatic coma. One should use this remedy with caution. If given in higher potency, it might bring the patient out of a merciful coma that precedes death.

PLUMBUM IODATUM. The remedy is used in the same way as *Opium,* but primarily for neurological, spinal, and head pains and for intracranial tumors *(see Chapter 2).* It also plays an important role in tumors growing from nerve cells and of the thyroid and pituitary glands.

The procedure for administering the above remedies is, roughly, as follows. The 30th or 200th potency is employed for as long as it is effective. When no longer effective, then one moves up the scale of dilutions. The appropriate remedy is given every hour, half-hour, fifteen, ten, or five minutes (or as often as needed) in water (stirring in between each dose if possible), ten times or until relief is obtained. Repeat procedure as often as is necessary—and change medicines as needed.

N.B. If the patient cannot swallow liquids, dry granules can be sprinkled into the mouth, or the lower lip can be pulled out and either wetted with liquid or sprinkled with a few granules.

Prototypal Case Example

A number of terminal cancer patients who have been treated by the Ramakrishnan method for at least six months will be able to profit from the "Plussing" method, without too frequent changes of remedies, up until the end. But some patients, especially those the homoeopathic practitioner inherits only in Stage IV, will need to have the medicines changed more frequently—sometimes more than once a day. The following case example is prototypal:

CASE 93   *September, 1999*

Female, 84 years, had a mastectomy of the right breast in 1996 and, because of her advanced years, opted not to undergo chemotherapy. For three years she did well and enthusiastically pursued her interests. In the spring of 1999, she was lacking her usual energy and was unable to garden. By early summer, she was experiencing some nausea and discomfort from eating. By July, she knew something was seriously wrong and underwent some tests to find out what was going on. Blood test results came back normal, but, against the recommendation of her oncologist, the patient decided not to have a CT scan at that time. At the end of September, the patient vomited blood, moved black stools, and went to the hospital.

> *An esophagogastroduodenoscopy (EGD) showed an ulcerated gastric mass in the proximal stomach. Bleeding was stopped with epinephrine injections. Biopsy confirmed the mass to be an adenocarcinoma. CT scan showed cancer, at Stage IV, had metastasized to the liver.*

With the supportive consent of her oncologist and surgeon, the patient chose not to combat the inevitable with surgery or chemotherapy but to work with homoeopathic remedies as much as possible until her demise.

PRESCRIPTION

September 29: *Phosphorus* 30C - several doses as a first aid treatment for internal bleeding

October 5:   At this point, treatment for the terminal stage commenced.

October-November:

> *Carcinosin* 30C - daily, single dose, before bed
> *Arsenicum album* 30C - single doses as needed for stomach pain and nausea
> *Chelidonium* 30C - single doses as needed for liver pain

> The patient did well managing her discomfort for two months. There was no sign of bleeding. Stools had returned to normal. She was able to eat small amounts at frequent intervals and continued with her normal daily activities.

December: As the patient's pain and discomfort increased, the potency of the pain-relieving remedies was raised to 200C and she began "plussing" the remedies, still taking them on an as-needed basis. Toward the end of December, the pain and discomfort became stronger. The patient could now only sip liquids and eat small pieces of fruit, and began occasionally to take a synthetic morphine along with the homoeopathic remedies. Sometimes she felt well, other times nauseated and experiencing malaise, but she continued to manage her affairs. During this month, on a couple of occasions, *Aconite* 30C was taken whenever the patient's anxiety, restlessness, and fear of death (taking the form of waves of panic attacks) prevented sleep at night (and *Arsenicum album* was ineffective).

January 1-7:   Although the narcotic was allowing periods of comfort, the need to increase the dosage soon set in. The patient's bowels stopped moving, her legs became swollen, and her mental clarity decreased. But until early January, she was still able to live alone and care for herself. At one point during this week, *Carcinosin* was discontinued so that she could concentrate on taking the more effective pain-relieving remedies, *Arsenicum* 200c and *Chelidonium* 200c.

January 8-11:   The patient was experiencing strong pain, and a full-time caretaker was required.
Arsenicum and *Chelidonium,* 1m potency in water, were taken frequently—as needed.
For two days during this time, *Scirrhinum* 200c - Split Dose Method, was administered for her liver pain when *Chelidonium* was no longer working. When *Scirrhinum* stopped working, *Chelidonium* 1m was returned to.

January 12:   Moved up to *Arsenicum album* 10m
Pain and nausea were not relieved and the patient was more impatient with her illness than usual. Nothing seemed to give her comfort; she was critical of her bed and insisted on moving to the sofa. And, above all, she was afraid that she would not be able to tolerate the pain any longer.
Nux vomica 200c - in water, taken as needed, gave physical relief, and the fear of the pain growing out of control was calmed.

January 13:   *Nux vomica* no longer effective in any potency.
Arsenicum album 200c was returned to with success.
Hydrastis 200c was now used instead of *Chelidonium* 1m.

The patient discontinued use of the narcotics. She preferred the continuous low level of discomfort with homoeopathic remedies to the high and low extremes experienced with narcotics. Her body functions improved and her mental clarity returned.

January 14:   *Hydrastis* had stopped working within 36 hours, and *Chelidonium* 1M was returned to, with good effect.

January 15-16: The narcotics no longer interfering, it became easier to observe the patient's symptoms and choose the appropriate remedy for them. When she, in discomfort, all of a sudden wanted water that was ice-cold rather than room temperature, *Phosphorus* took care of the discomfort immediately. *Phosphorus* was also given when fresh blood appeared in vomit, but *Cadmium sulphuratum* was used when blood in vomit looked like coffee grounds. *Sepia* 30C, one of the patient's regular constitutional remedies, was helpful when her nausea was accompanied by twitching in the inner thighs and her mood was despondent.

January 17:   *Arsenicum* 10M and *Chelidonium* 1M in water—frequently—alternating as needed.
Pain was relieved but the patient's restlessness continued to increase; instead of resting, she wanted to sit up and move around. Sleeping infrequently, it appeared as if she wanted to be awake when she died. At times the patient would only find relief in the classic *Arsenicum* position of sitting "with knees drawn up, resting her head and arms upon knees" (Kent). During this time she was still mentally alert and well capable of enjoying company.

> January 18:   The patient asked for the highest potency of *Arsenicum*. It was given to her in the 10M potency and she sank back into the pillows and began to reminisce. While talking, she experienced a strong pain in her liver, sat up to resume her *Arsenicum* position—and, within seconds, died.

If the homoeopathic practitioner is expecting to witness total relief from pain or discomfort, he might be disappointed. Sometimes the remedies can achieve this, but at other times, they can only help attain—and maintain—a relative degree of comfort and keep the pain down to a minimal or bearable level. Even here, however, it is still advisable, whenever possible, to pursue the homoeopathic remedies (changing remedies or potencies, as called for)—especially when the alternative is for a patient to take higher and higher dosages of painkillers and *still* experience pain; or when the pain returns with renewed force, after the painkiller wears off. Thus, a number of patients are most comfortable—and pass away more easily—if homoeopathic remedies are administered regularly alongside the painkillers.

The importance of having a caretaker committed to homoeopathy during the more advanced and/or terminal cancer stage cannot be overemphasized. There needs to be an objective person present to judge when and how often to administer the palliative medicines; also to observe when changes in potencies or remedies are needed. Often the caretaker can minimize pain by administering a dose of the appropriate remedy at the first sign of a decrease in the patient's comfort level (i.e., a change in the patient's facial expression or a restlessness of the body—it may be as subtle as furrowing of the brow or the twitching of a toe). Even if the patient appears to be asleep, the remedy can be administered to him in the manner noted on p. 166.

Of the several remedies to assist a patient during the final stage of his illness, the most frequently resorted to is *Arsenicum album* 10M. This remedy, administered on an as-needed basis (see Case 93), helps diminish the restlessness and pain, also the fear during the easing out ("Gives quiet and ease to the last moments of life when given in high potency": Boericke).

Other remedies that have proven of assistance during the period of relinquishing life are *Phosphorus, Lachesis,* and *Carbo vegetabilis* (according to the symptoms manifested). With these remedies, also, one might have to resort to the 1M, 10M, or 50M potencies.

Chapter 7
Classical Homoeopathy and the Ramakrishnan Method

The Place of Constitutional Prescribing in Cancer Treatment

It was noted in Chapter 1 that with cancer, when the practitioner so often finds himself in a race against time, a more aggressive form of treatment is required than with the majority of chronic diseases—and how even the cardinal homoeopathic tenet of "individualization" must give way before the "specificity" of the disease itself.

The Ramakrishnan Method, however, by no means precludes a homoeopath, well-versed in the classical approach, from employing his or her knowledge and skill whenever a patient's need for individualized constitutional treatment is perceived.* Indeed, as confirmed by numerous

---

*In a book of this nature full justice cannot be rendered to the question of constitutional prescribing. Those readers less familiar with the homoeopathic *materia medica* and the most commonly encountered "constitutional types," but who are seeking to learn more about these subjects, are advised to consult Boericke's *Materia Medica and Repertory* as the best beginning text and for an overall view. For more detailed descriptions of the physical and mental pictures of the remedies, Kent's *Lectures on the Materia Medica* or Margaret Tyler's *Homoeopathic Drug Pictures* are recommended. Finally, for those particularly interested in a more psychological approach and the interrelations between the mental-emotional and physical symptoms, Catherine R. Coulter's three-volume *Portraits of Homoeopathic Medicines* offers an in-depth psychophysical analysis of two dozen principal personality types (an abridged version of this last is found in *Nature and Human Personality: Homoeopathic Archetypes*). For all the above, see the Bibliography of Works Cited.

173

cases in the text, the two approaches ("constitutional" and "specific" prescribing) perfectly complement one another.

✦ Sometimes the constitutional remedy simply follows the cancer remedies, once the cancer is healed, contained, or controlled.

CASE 94   *February, 1995*

Female, 32 years, presented with a lump in the right breast, lower quadrant. It was stony hard, freely mobile, measuring 1 inch in diameter, and painless. There was no adenitis.

> *Biopsy report: Adenocarcinoma, Stage I. Contrary to advice, the patient refused surgery and wanted only homoeopathy.*

The woman was a typical *Pulsatilla:* of a mild, yielding, obliging disposition, sociable, and, because of her innate indecisiveness, liking others to take over; yet at the same time, possessing a stubborn streak, as witnessed in her refusal—against all advice—to undergo surgery.

PRESCRIPTION

Week 1:	*Conium* 200c - daily, Plussing Method
Week 2:	*Scirrhinum* 200c - daily, Plussing Method
Weeks 3-8:	Same as Weeks 1-2 Lump was significantly softer and smaller.
Weeks 9-12:	Same as Weeks 1-2 Lump remained softer and smaller, and Dr. Ramakrishnan judged it time to try the constitutional remedy.
Week 13:	*Pulsatilla* 200c† - daily, Plussing Method Lump completely gone.
Week 14:	*Scirrhinum* 200c - daily, Plussing Method
Weeks 15-28:	Same as Weeks 13-14

Mammogram indicated no lump.

Months 8-10: Same as Weeks 13-14, but in the 1M potency

Months 11-16: *Pulsatilla* 1M and *Scirrhinum* 1M - alternating semimonthly, Split Dose Method

For the next year: Same as Months 11-16, but in the 10M potency

> *For five years now, tests have shown the patient to be free of cancer.*

REMARKS

This case clearly shows the use of an organ-specific remedy *(Conium)*, the appropriate nosode *(Scirrhinum)*, and the constitutional remedy *(Pulsatilla)* working in concert.

✦ At other times, the constitutional remedy (or remedies) will be administered to assist the stymied cancer nosode and/or organ-specific remedy.

CASE 95   *September, 1997*

Female, 38 years, presented with a cancerous bony growth in the upper end of the right tibia, Stage II.

> *History: A diagnosed osteoclastoma in the tibia was operated on in June, 1996; no chemotherapy or radiation therapy was done. In June, 1997, there was a recurrence in the same place, which was again surgically treated. In August, 1997, there was a second recurrence and the patient turned to homoeopathy.*

The woman was constipated and overweight, with poor physical stamina and a tendency to perspire upon the least exertion, prone to bone spurs. She was full of original ideas, restless to execute them but, in actuality, a plodder—all symptoms suggestive of *Calcarea carbonica*. Additionally, a strong tubercular heredity in her case history pointed to *Tuberculinum*.

PRESCRIPTION

Week 1:   *Hekla lava* 200c - daily, Plussing Method

Week 2:   *Carcinosin* 200c - daily, Plussing Method

Weeks 3-8:   Same as Weeks 1-2
               Size of the tumor was reduced by 25%.

Weeks 9-16:   Same as Weeks 1-8
               Tumor slightly smaller, but not significantly so, and not enough to continue with the same remedies.

Week 17:   *Calcarea carbonica* 200c† - daily, Plussing Method

Week 18:   *Tuberculinum bovinum* 200c - daily, Plussing Method
               Improvement was more marked.

Weeks 19-24:   Same as Weeks 17-18
               With these two remedies, the tumor was reduced by another 50% to 60%.

Months 7-9:   Same as Weeks 17-18
               Size of the tumor remained the same.

Months 10-12: *Hekla lava* 1M and *Carcinosin* 1M, alternating weekly - daily, Plussing Method
               Tumor was down to 10% of its original size.

For two more years, the woman has continued to take the two remedies in the 10M potency, alternating monthly, Split Dose Method. Today, the lump is still 10% of its original size and the patient is doing well.

Periodic CT scans show condition stable.

✦ Likewise, the constitutional remedy can be brought in when there is metastasis after an apparent cure.

CASE 96   *July, 1994*

Male child, 12 years, was brought in with a 6 cm. Ewing's sarcoma of the left fibula, Stage II.

> *Radiation and chemotherapy advised, but parents refused and turned to homoeopathy.*

The boy was fine-featured, bright, chirpy, extroverted, overactive, with a fear of animals—a typical *Tuberculinum* child. One of his parents had had tuberculosis.

PRESCRIPTION

Week 1:   *Hekla lava* 200c - daily, Plussing Method

Week 2:   *Carcinosin* 200c - daily, Plussing Method

Weeks 3-30:   Same as Weeks 1-2
                        In six months the tumor was completely gone.

> *In the beginning of March, 1995, a routine CT scan picked up an area of metastasis in the right ankle—the lateral malleolus.*

Weeks 31-42: *Tuberculinum bovinum* 10M† - weekly, Split Dose Method

> *CT scan in June showed no lesions.*

Thereafter, and to date, *Tuberculinum bovinum* 10M has been prescribed once or twice a year as a preventive measure.

REMARKS

As can be observed in this and other examples (Cases 43, 62, 77, and 95), Dr. Ramakrishnan is inclined to employ *Tuberculinum* when there is a patient or family history of tuberculosis. Here, the choice of remedy was accentuated by the boy's constitutional type.

For the short duration of the Plussing and Split Dose Method, see *N.B.* after Case 59.

✦ Occasionally, in the earlier stages of the disease, the patient's constitutional medicine can be prescribed from the beginning, in alternation with a cancer nosode or a wide-spectrum cancer specific. It is especially appropriate if the remedy has an affinity with the site of the tumor or the organ involved. This procedure has been encountered repeatedly in these pages, and the following is merely an additional illustration.

CASE 97   *August, 1994*

Female, 29 years, presented with an ulcer on the left vocal cord and hoarseness. No submandibular or cervical glands were palpable and the larynx looked healthy.

> *Tissue from the ulcer underwent histopathological examination; the diagnosis was squamous cell carcinoma, Stage I. The patient refused radiation therapy.*

The woman displayed *Phosphorus* characteristics. She was pretty, bright-eyed, and artistic: fond of books and music, exhibiting skills in weaving, embroidery, etc. She also exhibited a fear of the dark and of strangers. Her food preferences were for sour, salt, and for cold drinks.

PRESCRIPTION

Week 1:   *Phosphorus* 200c† - daily, Plussing Method

Week 2:   *Carcinosin* 200c - daily, Plussing Method

> *Laryngoscopic examination showed improvement in appearance of the ulcer and more mobility.*

Weeks 3-8:   Same as Weeks 1-2

Laryngoscopy was performed every two weeks and a CT scan after seven weeks. At the end of eight weeks, tests showed that the vocal cord was healed and the patient's voice was normal.

Months 3-4:   Same as Weeks 1-2

At the end of sixteen weeks, the oncologist pronounced the patient out of danger.

Month 5:   *Phosphorus* 1M - once, Split Dose Method

Month 6:   *Carcinosin* 1M - once, Split Dose Method

Months 7-8:   Same as Months 5-6

Thereafter, *Carcinosin* 1M - quarterly for approximately two years, Split Dose Method.

After one year, a laryngoscopy was performed and everything continued to show clear.

✦ Opening a case with the constitutional remedy is frequently employed in cancers of the female reproductive system, when one of the classic "female" remedies *(Pulsatilla, Sepia, Lachesis, Lilium tigrinum)* is indicated. The following case exemplifies this point:

CASE 98   *January, 1996*

Female, 37 years, presented with a lump in the right breast, upper quadrant, which, over the last three years, despite treatment with another type of alternative therapy, had grown from 0.5 to 2 cm. in diameter. The cancerous mass was hard, but still mobile, Stage II.

The original biopsy revealed an infiltrating ductile carcinoma. An examination of both breasts and the axillae and an ultrasonogram showed no other lumps or abnormal glands. A full-body CT scan (because three years had elapsed, during which time there could have been metastasis) showed everything clear.

The woman was dyspeptic, with a sinking feeling in the stomach and sometimes a burning pain on eructation; also soreness in the abdomen. She was clever, rising fast in the business world, and highly independent; rather stern upon first acquaintance and wary of too-close relationships, but good company once she dropped her reserve.

PRESCRIPTION

Week 1:   *Sepia* 200c† - daily, Plussing Method

Week 2:   *Scirrhinum* 200c - daily, Plussing Method

Weeks 3-4:   Same as Weeks 1-2
               Some improvement discernible in the nature of the lump.

Month 2:   Same as Weeks 1-2
               A substantial reduction in the size of the tumor was discernible.

Months 3-6:   Same as Weeks 1-2
               Improvement continued.

Months 7-12:   Same as Weeks 1-2, but in the 1M potency
               Size of lump reduced still further to 0.5 cm.

Months 13-16: Same as Months 7-12
               Condition stable, with perhaps a slight improvement.

Months 17-22: Same as Months 7-12, but in the 10M potency
               Lump completely disappeared.

For the next year, the patient received one dose of *Sepia* 10M and *Scirrhinum* 10M, alternating monthly, Split Dose Method. She is no longer receiving any remedies and continues to be healthy.

✦ In the following case one observes that no cancer nosode was employed at all. But then, usually an organ-specific remedy, or a remedy highly specific to the site of the tumor, or some other nosode will be prescribed together with the constitutional remedy.

CASE 99 [p-P]   *May, 1987*

Male, 53 years, presented with rectal bleeding and a 4 cm. cauliflower growth in the rectum.

> *Colonoscopy revealed the ascending, transverse, and descending colon to be entirely clear. Results of CT scan of all abdominal organs and lungs also were negative. Diagnosed as an adenocarcinoma, Stage I.*

Typical of *Silica,* the patient was conscientious in everything he undertook and competent, but he was shy and lacking in self-confidence. Physically, he was intolerant of cold drafts, especially to the head and sinuses, and suffered from lingering skin infections, particularly around the nails.

PRESCRIPTION

Month 1:   *Silica* 200c† - weekly, Split Dose Method
                A little progress.

Month 2:   *Thuja* 200c - weekly, Split Dose Method
                More improvement.

Months 3-6:   Same as Months 1-2
                The patient was much improved.

Months 7-9:   Same as Months 1-2
                The entire mass had disappeared.

> *The rectum was examined by proctoscope, and a subsequent colonoscopy showed everything clear.*

For eighteen months, the patient continued to receive the same two remedies in monthly alternations, Split Dose Method. Thereafter, he was given *Silica* 1M, his constitutional remedy, quarterly,

Split Dose Method. This prescription continues to date as a preventative.

REMARKS

In this case, *Thuja,* acting as an organ-specific remedy, apparently obviated the necessity of a cancer nosode, although today Dr. Ramakrishnan would probably have alternated *Thuja* with one of the latter.

✦ On certain occasions, especially in the earlier stages and with slow-growing tumors such as those of the thyroid, a case can be handled solely with periodic constitutional and acute remedies.

CASE 100   *September, 1997*

Female, 49 years, cancer of the thyroid. After the removal of her left thyroid lobe, which was diagnosed as cancerous, her oncologist wanted to remove the right half, in which there were signs of nodular growths. Scans showed the lobe to be misshapen, and the patient's serum thyroglobulin levels were elevated (suggesting residual thyroid cancer). The patient refused to undergo this procedure and chose instead the homoeopathic route. The oncologist agreed to a nine-month trial, provided she was monitored regularly. The woman would receive a remedy every month to six weeks, as her physical and mental symptoms dictated: starting with *Thuja* 1M for her constitutional picture—fortuitously (but at that time unbeknownst to the prescriber) the preeminent remedy for thyroid cancer; then moving on to *Natrum muriaticum* 10M when she was experiencing much grief from a heartbreak; then *Sepia* 1M for protracted dejection and low self-esteem, better from vigorous exercise; then repeated doses of *Phosphorus* 200c as an acute remedy for her recurring sore throats with loss of voice, and *Spongia* if these developed into a recalcitrant cough; then back to *Thuja* 1M again whenever she experienced loss of confidence in or, especially, fear of her work (she was a psychic by profession). After the second three-month sonogram, the growths were smaller and, after the third, the shape of the thyroid lobe was beginning to look normal. She continued regular homoeopathic treatment, and after eighteen months her thyroid lobe looked completely healthy, with no alarming signs of any nodules or growths—and all tests continue normal to date.

A number of cases, then, have, over the decades, been successfully treated by the classical method alone, but this requires more experience and expertise than the average homoeopath possesses. Moreover, regardless of how dramatic or sensational the results, the cases are *so* individual as to be of little teaching value. The remedies that helped one patient will not necessarily help another, even with a highly similar condition. Additionally, in urgent or more advanced cases, the constitutional approach is insufficient, and many practitioners have found themselves grateful for the tried and proven rules and procedures offered in these pages. Even the more experienced homoeopath can enhance his skills by an effective combination of the constitutional approach and the Ramakrishnan Method.

Treatment of Acute Ailments During the Plussing Method

A procedural point necessary to address is that of prescribing remedies for intercurrent acute conditions that arise during the treatment of cancer. How are the acute remedies to be managed so as not to interfere with the Plussing Method?

✦ In acute conditions (such as a bodily injury, high fever, or a bout of influenza) the Plussing Method is *not* discontinued. The appropriate acute remedy is sometimes prescribed in the 30c or lower potency (so as to interfere less with the 200c medicines), in a way that works around the two- to three-hour "plussing" time—in the same way that allopathic medications (digitalis or nitroglycerin for heart, anticonvulsive drugs for seizures, or insulin for diabetes) are timed so as not to coincide with the cancer remedies.

✦ If the condition is a hemorrhage or excessive bleeding from the tumor itself or around the site of the tumor, *Phosphorus* and *Sanguinaria* are the preferred remedies (*see Chapter 2* and Cases 14, 30, 75, and 91). In these instances, which can be life-threatening, the cancer remedies are suspended for as long as *Phosphorus* or *Sanguinaria* are called for.

✦ Once a case has stabilized and the cancer is improving or under control, the practitioner can concentrate on the acute condition before returning to his "cancer" regimen.

CASE 101 [p-P]   *February, 1993*

Male, 58 years, presented with a five-year history of recurring hematuria (blood in urine).

> *Cystoscopic findings revealed a huge cauliflower-like growth. Biopsy report: Adenocarcinoma of the bladder, Stage III. The patient turned to homoeopathy.*

PRESCRIPTION

Weeks 1-4:   *Terebinthina* 200c - daily, Plussing Method

Week 5:   *Carcinosin* 200c - daily, Plussing Method

Weeks 6-14:   Same as Weeks 1-5

> *Cystoscopy revealed the mass to be substantially smaller.*

But the patient had a peptic ulcer, with the typical *Sulphur* 11 a.m. to 12:00 noon aggravation. This had to be addressed.

Weeks 15-19:   *Sulphur* 200c - daily, Plussing Method
               Peptic ulcer was much improved, but not resolved.

Weeks 20-23:   *Carcinosin* 200c resumed - daily, Plussing Method

> *Cystoscopy showed further resolution of the mass.*

But ulcer symptoms still not entirely resolved.

Weeks 24-27:   *Sulphur* 200c - daily, Plussing Method
               The patient was asymptomatic.

The patient then ceased his visits. He returned after three years, still asymptomatic and doing well.

Follow-up cystoscopy showed the same as after Weeks 20-23.

PRESCRIPTION

Week 1:   *Terebinthina* 200c - once, Split Dose Method (because the patient refused to be "shackled" by having to take remedies more than once a week)

Week 2:   *Carcinosin* 200c - once, Split Dose Method

Weeks 3-24:   Same as Weeks 1-2

Cystoscopy showed no trace of the mass.

The patient again dropped out of sight for two years, but when he returned, he was put on the same regimen as Weeks 1-2 for six months. Then the patient stopped coming *again*. This on-and-off pattern continues to this day. (No further tests given.)

REMARKS

See also Case 111—an even clearer illustration of interrupting the Plussing Method in order to treat an acute condition.

✦ Sometimes even an acute mental condition can be addressed, while the "cancer" remedies are postponed—since the mental symptoms are often prime indicators of the always helpful constitutional remedy. If this last proves helpful for the cancer as well, it can be continued, alternating with a cancer nosode.

CASE 102   *April, 1993*

Male, 43 years, presented with a pancreatic cancer, Stage III. He was experiencing abdominal pain, jaundice, and severe vomiting (first occurrence was early in 1993). He was very weak, very cold, had lost 50 lb. in three months, and was periodically vomiting black, coffee-ground-like matter.

Tests showed bilirubin 23 mg./dL.; liver enzyme levels, SGOT/SGPT, were 180 and 155; blood sugar was 240 mg. Surgery was performed, and a huge mass was found at the head of the pancreas, pressing on the duodenum, bile duct, and ampulla of Vater. Only two-thirds of the mass could be removed.

PRESCRIPTION

Week 1:   *Cadmium sulphuratum* 200c - daily, Plussing Method

Week 2:   *Carcinosin* 200c - daily, Plussing Method
The patient felt much better.

Weeks 3-10:   Same as Weeks 1-2
The patient continued to improve clinically. He had gained 10 lb. and had not vomited for four weeks.

CT scan showed no change.

Weeks 11-15: *Carcinosin* 200c - daily, Plussing Method
At this point, the patient's picture changed. He became more fearful, was restless, and his complaints took on a burning character.

Weeks 16-20: *Arsenicum album* 200c - daily, Plussing Method
The patient improved still further in his well-being and looked much healthier.

CT scan showed that the mass in the abdomen remained the same.

For eighteen months, the patient received *Arsenicum album* 200c and *Carcinosin* 200c—alternating weekly, Split Dose Method.

CT scan showed no change.

Seven years later, still on the same two remedies, but now in the 1M potency alternating monthly, the patient continues well and is able to do about three hours of gentle work daily. He eats well and digests well. But the CT scan shows the mass in the abdomen remains the same, so the patient is not yet out of danger.

REMARKS

Cadmium sulphuratum was originally prescribed on the basis of the patient's extreme chilliness and weakness, the black, coffee-ground-like vomit, and, as noted earlier, because it is one of the finest organ-specific remedies for stomach and pancreatic cancer *(see Chapter 2).*

Another example of *Arsenicum album* "taking over" is found in Case 117.

In sum, although in his treatment of cancer Dr. Ramakrishnan has primarily developed and refined the "specific" approach, he will, when necessary, at any given point during treatment, employ the acute or the constitutional approach.

The Potencies

As can be observed in virtually all of the case examples cited in this book, the 200C is the preferred potency in the Ramakrishnan Method of treating cancer. At times, however—especially when dealing with terminal or geriatric cases, or with those patients who are hypersensitive to the homoeopathic dilutions or who are in a delicate, precarious state—starting with, or dropping down to, the 30th potency (whether 30X or 30C is immaterial) might achieve better results.

CASE 103 [p-P]   *June, 1992*

Male child, 6 years, was brought in with severe anemia, a bloated abdomen, and enlarged spleen and liver. There was a severe tendency to hemorrhage; every day he would bleed from somewhere (either from the lungs, vomit blood, or have blood in the urine or conjunctiva) and would become extremely weak.

Diagnosed myelogenous leukemia, Stage IV.

PRESCRIPTION

Week 1:   *China* 30C - hourly, ten times a day

	Bleeding stopped for five days. A little blood in the urine on Day 6.
Week 2:	Same as Week 1 No bleeding for one week.
Week 3:	*Calcarea carbonica* 200c - once, Split Dose Method Condition stable.*
Week 4:	Same as Week 3 Condition stable.

Since the boy was in Stage IV, during the next two months many remedies (*Aconite, Arsenicum album, Kali carbonica,* and *Sanguinaria*) were given on an as-needed basis (see Case 93). He seemingly made a dramatic recovery—condition continued stable. But during the fifth month of treatment, there was suddenly a massive hemorrhage in the lungs and the boy died that day.

REMARKS

During the four months of homoeopathic treatment, the boy felt strong and happy. No bleeding episodes. *China* is an important remedy when there is extreme weakness from loss of body fluids.

Calcarea carbonica was prescribed because the remedy is so often required by (and is beneficial for) children.

---

*Here again, in this case and in the pre-Plussing ones that follow, today Dr. Ramakrishnan would have used the Plussing Method and a cancer nosode for better results.

✦ Certain remedies are prescribed in low potency for intercurrent ailments and infections that arise during the treatment of cancer and are related to the disease. *Arsenicum iodatum,* for instance, is of benefit to patients susceptible to repeated infections in or around the site of the tumor—and is interpolated with the cancer remedies.

CASE 104 [p-P]   *January, 1989*

> Female, 40 years, presented with a huge neglected cancerous mass in right breast, now, obviously at Stage IV. The open wound was septic, with a sloughing base, everted margins, and a copious, bloodstained discharge. The numerous axillary glands were big and coalesced. Pain was deep-seated: burning, stinging, and pulling.
>
> > *Since the case was terminal, the patient's doctor saw no point to subjecting her to any tests.*
>
> The woman was of a sensitive, lachrymose disposition, and craved sympathy and support. Physically, she was thirstless, better from motion and in the open air, and her pains tended to wander from one part of the body to another.

PRESCRIPTION

> Weeks 1-4: *Phytolacca* 200C - daily, Split Dose Method
> Also, *Arsenicum iodatum* 6X - daily, two tablets four times a day
> The discharge stopped completely. The wound shrunk a little and showed signs of healing. Pain relief was significant.
>
> Week 5: *Pulsatilla* 200C† - daily, Split Dose Method
> *Arsenicum iodatum* 6X - continued daily
>
> Week 6: *Phytolacca* 200C - daily, Split Dose Method
> *Arsenicum iodatum* 6X - continued daily
>
> Weeks 7-8: Same as Weeks 5-6
> The patient continued comfortable. Condition stable.

Month 3:   Same as Weeks 5-6

During the fourth month, there was a severe hemorrhage from the wound, which could not be controlled either by homoeopathic or allopathic medicines. The woman was hospitalized and died four days later.

REMARKS

Phytolacca was the most appropriate organ-specific remedy, *Pulsatilla* the constitutional one.

See also Cases 5, 64, 70, 118, and 119 for the concomitant use of low-potency *Arsenicum iodatum* with cancer remedies.

The Schuessler Cell Salt *Calcarea fluorica* is often prescribed concomitantly with other remedies for cancers of the bone (see Cases 116 and 121). In general, the Schuessler Cell Salts, prescribed in low potency, have proven to be effective supportive measures *(see Chapter 9)*.

The tinctures *Ornithogalum* and *Chelidonium*, always taken in water *(see Chapter 2)* and sipped as often as needed for symptom relief, can be taken concomitantly with the cancer remedies—although not at exactly the same time of the day (see Cases 32 and 105).

The more frequently encountered question of when to *increase* the strength of a medicine (when to "raise the potency") is determined in part by the rate of progress, in part by intuition born of experience, and therefore lends itself to no definite rules. However, Dr. Ramakrishnan does offer some general guidelines.

✦ As long as a patient is progressing, the prescriber continues with the 200c potency, reevaluating the case every four to six (or eight) weeks.

✦ If improvement ceases or has reached a plateau, when one expects better results or when the rate of progress is not as satisfying or as marked as it used to be, this might be an indication to move up the scale of dilutions.

CASE 105 [p-P]   *November, 1980*

Male, 52 years, reported with a diagnosed cancer of the stomach, Stage IV. Symptoms were persistent nausea, extreme weakness, and total inability to take any solids.

> *Endoscopy revealed a mass the size of a lemon in the higher fundus of stomach, almost blocking the cardiac orifice. The entire mucous membrane was strewn with ulcerations. Biopsy report: Adenocarcinoma; CT scan revealed involvement of the liver and spleen. The patient did not want any Western medication or procedures and turned to homoeopathy.*

The patient had always been fearful and impulsive. He had a strong craving for both sweets and salt (but with symptoms aggravated by sugar); he was significantly better in the open, fresh (even cold) air and his lifelong digestive complaints (gnawings, burnings, painful swellings) had always been better from strong pressure on the stomach. All symptoms were suggestive of *Argentum nitricum*.

PRESCRIPTION

Weeks 1-6:   *Argentum nitricum* 200C† - weekly, Split Dose Method
Also *Ornithogalum* ø in water - sip taken as needed, at least several times a day
The patient felt better, then plateaued.

Weeks 7-10:   Same as Week 1, but in the 1M potency
Progress continued slowly, then plateaued again.

Weeks 11-14:   Same as Week 1, but in the 10M potency
The patient improved a bit more, then remained stable.

Thereafter, and for nine months until his death, the patient would receive periodic doses of *Argentum nitricum* 10M.

REMARKS

Argentum nitricum was the perfect constitutional remedy. But it can also be an excellent remedy for stomach cancer.

The soothing effects of *Ornithogalum* ø in stomach cancer cannot be overestimated *(see Chapter 2)*.

✦ If there are signs of relapse or recurrence, the potency may be raised.

CASE 106 [p-P]   *April, 1991*

Female, 47 years, who was a long-time tobacco-chewer, presented with a diagnosed squamous cell carcinoma of the right cheek, Stage II. Her symptoms were a foul odor from the mouth, with a putrid discharge from the ulcer and a flabby tongue.

The woman was from a small Indian village and had neglected the ulcer until it had reached at least Stage II. She also had a tendency to dyspepsia with a sinking feeling in the stomach around 12:00 noon, perspired freely, and was always hot. She was careless of her hygiene, and the body tended to emit odors.

PRESCRIPTION

Week 1:   *Hydrastis* 200C - daily, Split Dose Method
               Tobacco-chewing was discontinued from day one.

Weeks 2-12:   Same as Week 1
               Ulcer 75% improved and the submandibular gland almost gone. At this point, the patient stopped coming.

In April, 1992, the woman returned to report that the remedy had worked remarkably well, with 90% of symptoms cleared, but that during the last two months, there were signs of recurrence.

PRESCRIPTION

Months 1-8:   *Hydrastis* 1M - semimonthly, Split Dose Method
               Symptoms cleared again.

Months 9-21:   *Sulphur* 200c† - semimonthly, Split Dose Method
The lesion was completely healed and the patient remains healthy to date.

REMARKS

Hydrastis was chosen because of the patient's large, flabby tongue and for this remedy's affinity for ulcerations of any part of the alimentary canal, especially between the mouth and stomach.

Sulphur was selected after *Hydrastis* had done its specific work because of the woman's general symptoms and constitutional picture.

✦ On the other hand (and this is where intuition enters the picture), at times the physician will choose to move up the scale of dilutions simply to hasten the healing process. The following is one of many such instances found in this book:

CASE 107   *January, 1994*

Male, 72 years, who had been a heavy smoker for 30 years, sought homoeopathic assistance for a severe cough with bloodstained expectoration. He was diagnosed as having bronchogenic cancer, Stage III.

> *History: A left lobectomy had been performed in 1992. In September, 1993, there was a recurrence in the lower right lobe. This was operated on— after which the patient turned to homoeopathy.*

Other symptoms were short, jerky breathing; sharp, cutting pain in the chest, radiating either down into the stomach or up into the shoulder; even the slightest cough or exertion produced severe dyspnea and cyanosis.

PRESCRIPTION

Week 1:   *Oxalicum acidum* 200c - daily, Plussing Method

Week 2:   *Scirrhinum* 200c - daily, Plussing Method
                 Some improvement.

Weeks 3-4:   Same as Weeks 1-2
                 There was tremendous relief of all symptoms: no
                 cough, less breathlessness, no cyanosis. Also, the
                 patient looked much healthier.

Months 2-3:   Same as Weeks 1-2
                 Improvement continued but, nevertheless, the
                 doctor decided to raise the potency.

Months 4-5:   Same as Weeks 1-2, but in the 1M potency
                 The patient was feeling completely well.

Thereafter, the patient received *Oxalicum acidum* 1M and *Scirrhinum* 1M, alternating, semimonthly, Split Dose Method— and continues, to this day, to do well on this regimen.

REMARKS

Oxalicum acidum was prescribed on the basis of the specific symptoms described above.

Scirrhinum was selected over *Carcinosin* because the operation procedure and summary reported that the mass in the lobe of the lung was rock hard.

✦ A final point: in advanced or terminal cases, a frequent *alternation of the potencies* of the remedies employed (moving both up and down the scale) is sometimes required, either to address the condition on different levels or to ensure that the patient does not tire of, and cease to respond to, a particular potency (see Case 93). This situation arises when the Plussing Method no longer works and when the practitioner, no longer striving for healing, is concerned only with palliation.

Chapter 8
Homoeopathy and Western Medicine

Homoeopathy works highly effectively in conjunction with a number of Western medical procedures. In fact, the majority of cancer patients seeking homoeopathic assistance have already undergone, are undergoing, or are about to undergo some form of allopathic treatment—and entertain hopes that the two forms of medicine can work well together. As a rule, this partnership presents few problems.*

As can be observed in the numerous cases cited in earlier chapters, far from minimizing the usefulness of Western diagnostic tests and routine follow-up procedures (and even certain methods of treating the cancer), the homoeopath views these as highly important. With the information gleaned from them, he can better understand a patient's condition and regulate the homoeopathic prescriptions accordingly. For this reason, every homoeopathic cancer patient is urged and encouraged, for his own well-being, to find an oncologist willing to cooperate and work with a homoeopathic doctor.

---

*The question of homoeopathy's working in conjunction with alternative (nonconventional) therapies is addressed in the Appendix, Question 20.

Surgery

Dr. Ramakrishnan generally recommends surgery, even in the early stages of the disease when the lump or primary tumor is small, before it is fixed or crowding and impinging on the surrounding organs, causing pain and discomfort, and before it is too late to operate. Excision of such a tumor (and when possible, the secondary lesions, such as the axillary or mesenteric glands) not only brings physical relief, but also delays (if only temporarily) the cancer's spread to other organs—thus buying time. Because *homoeopathy achieves its healing effects by counteracting the body's propensity to form tumors,* additional time to allow the homoeopathic remedies to take effect is crucial. In short, when the tumor or the affected lymph glands are still operable, *surgery, followed by homoeopathy is, in Dr. Ramakrishnan's opinion, the optimal procedure.*

The trauma of surgical procedures can be lessened substantially and the healing process accelerated in the following ways:

✦ *Presurgical care: Arnica* 200C potency—administered twice, once on the day before and a second time just prior to surgery—prepares the soft tissue cells for the shock of incisions.

✦ For *fear of upcoming surgery, Aconite* 200C can be administered the night before—and then repeated, if necessary, an hour or two prior to surgery. In a highly anxious patient whose fears do not respond to *Aconite, Arsenicum album* 200C can be prescribed instead of *Aconite.*

✦ *Postsurgical care: Arnica* 200C, administered four times a day (or as often as needed) for at least one week after surgery. This remedy can be alternated with *Hypericum* 200C if there is much pain, and at times there may be a need to move up to the higher potencies of these two remedies to obtain the desired relief. Additionally, *Hypericum* is especially useful after head surgery when there are postsurgical complications, including seizures.

CASE 108   *June, 1994*

Male, 25 years, reported with seizures following surgery for brain cancer. Diagnosis was glioma, Stage II.

> *History: After six months of headaches, a CT scan revealed a mass in the left parietal zone. Surgery was performed, and the histopathological report confirmed glioma. Radiation treatment followed. But soon after, the patient started having seizures.*

PRESCRIPTION

Week 1:   *Hypericum* 200C - daily, Plussing Method

Week 2:   *Carcinosin* 200C - daily, Plussing Method
               The seizures stopped.

Weeks 3-16:   Same as Weeks 1-2
               The patient was feeling well.

> *CT scan showed a recurrence of growth in the same area. Since the lesion was still too small for surgery, the surgeon decided to wait until it was larger.*

Week 17:   *Plumbum iodatum* 200C - daily, Plussing Method

Week 18:   *Carcinosin* 200C - daily, Plussing Method

Weeks 19-24:   Same as Weeks 17-18

> *Scan showed the tumor to be the same size.*

Months 7-8:   Same as Weeks 17-18

> *Scan showed that the tumor was gone.*

Months 9-18:   Same remedies as during Weeks 17-18, but alternating semimonthly, Split Dose Method

Thereafter, the patient received periodic doses of either remedy and has remained healthy to date.

REMARKS

The value of *Plumbum iodatum* in brain tumors was discussed in Chapter 2.

Another remedy to consider in the event that *Arnica* is not helping is *Bellis perennis*. Indeed, some doctors even give preference to this remedy for injury to the deeper tissues (which includes major surgery, especially to the breast).

✦ *Postoperative bleeding: Phosphorus,* with its picture of hemorrhaging *(see Chapters 2 and 7)* is the principal remedy for excessive or unarrestable postoperative bleeding. In patients who are susceptible to excessive bleeding, the remedy can be administered prior to surgery instead of *Arnica* (in which case, the latter would have been given a few hours earlier). *Lachesis* and *Sanguinaria* are other remedies for postoperative hemorrhage when *Phosphorus* is not effective.

✦ If the patient experiences *painful postsurgical incarceration of flatus,* the best remedy is *Carbo vegetabilis* 30c, administered as called for.

✦ In cases of *postsurgical adhesions* and *excessive scar tissue* causing pain or other symptoms, the best remedies are *Graphites* and *Causticum*. An example of each follows.

CASE 109   *March, 1997*

Female, 37 years, who had been operated on three times within the preceding nine months for ovarian cancer, had then to undergo three laparoscopic surgeries to remove adhesions that were causing unbearable pain. Six surgical procedures in two years and, once again, recurring adhesions brought her to homoeopathy.

> *CT scans, blood tests, and physical examinations showed her to be clear of malignancy at the moment.*

PRESCRIPTION

Month 1:   *Graphites* 200c - weekly, Split Dose Method
                 Also, *Colocynthis* 200c - every five minutes, ten
                 times whenever acute colicky pains were experi-
                 enced.

Months 2-4:   Same as Weeks 1-4
                 The patient felt 50% better.

Months 5-12:   Same as Weeks 1-4
                 Pain entirely disappeared.

During this time, the patient was also prescribed, constitutionally, monthly doses of *Pulsatilla* 200c, Split Dose Method.

Thereafter, the patient has periodically kept in touch with the doctor and is doing well.

CASE 110   *June, 1997*

Female, 43 years, presented after undergoing an operation for ovarian cancer, Stage II. She was experiencing severe abdominal pain, which did not respond to any painkiller. CT scan did not reveal anything. Colonoscopy, upper GI endoscopy, and other tests showed everything normal.

> *History: The patient had had three cesarean sections, an appendectomy, and six months previously an ovarian cancer operated on—followed by chemotherapy. A recent laparotomy to investigate the cause of pain revealed adhesions.*

PRESCRIPTION

Week 1:   *Causticum* 200c - daily, Plussing Method

Week 2:   *Carcinosin* 200c - daily, Plussing Method
                 The patient experienced almost instant relief.

Weeks 3-14:   Same as Weeks 1-2
                 Pain entirely gone.

Weeks 15-26:   For preventive purposes, the patient was kept on these two remedies, but in the 1M potency

That was the end of treatment, and the woman continues healthy.

REMARKS

Causticum was selected rather than *Graphites* because of the evidence of spasm of the colon and irregular bowels.

For additional examples of postsurgical adhesions or fibrosis, see Cases 22 and 84.

✦ *If the surgical incision (especially an incision in the abdominal cavity) is not healing well,* the preferred remedy is *Staphysagria* 200C—to be administered as needed.

✦ *Staphysagria* is also the preferred remedy for *postsurgical urethral strictures.* This remedy will often obviate the need of a catheter.

CASE 111   *June, 1995*

Male, 62 years, presented with a biopsy-confirmed adenocarcinoma of the prostate, Stage II, which he had chosen to have treated with homoeopathy. Symptoms were weak flow of urine and a PSA level of 22.

PRESCRIPTION

Week 1:   *Conium* 200C - daily, Plussing Method

Week 2:   *Carcinosin* 200C - daily, Plussing Method

Weeks 3-8:   Same as Weeks 1-2
               The flow of urine was stronger and there was no urgency. PSA level dropped to 16.

Weeks 9-16:   Same as Weeks 1-2
               The patient continued to improve.

               CT scan confirmed the surgeon's observation (upon palpation) that the gland had become smaller and softer.

At this point, the patient developed a stricture in the urethra. He had had this condition several times before, as a result of a history of recurrent cystitis (50 to 60 times), for which he was prescribed antibiotics. The strictures had required urethral dilations.

Week 17:   *Staphysagria* 200c - daily, Split Dose Method
After six to eight hours, there was a tremendous relief from pain over the bladder, which had been due to acute retention of urine. After three days, the condition was resolved.

Weeks 18-32:   Same as Weeks 1-2
By the eighth month, everything cleared; both the cancer and the episodes of stricture of the urethra were resolved.

Months 9-16:   Same as Weeks 1-2, but in the 1M potency and alternating semimonthly, Split Dose Method

Months 17-24:   Same as Weeks 1-2, but in the 10M potency, alternating monthly, Split Dose Method

> *Between Months 8 and 24, the PSA level had steadily dropped to 3.2, where it remains to this day.*

End of treatment.

REMARKS

Carcinosin was selected over *Scirrhinum* because of a strong cancer heredity.

If *Staphysagria* does not work, *Sepia* (contrary to expectation, primarily in males) or *Causticum* (for either gender) might be effective.

✦ *Terebinthina* has proven effective for *urinary incontinence follow-ing surgery of the prostate.*

CASE 112   *April, 1994*

Male, 82 years, presented with symptoms of frequency of micturi-tion, passing in dribbles and with considerable pain (strangury), and bloodstained urine.

> *Biopsy revealed an adenocarcinoma of the prostate, Stage II. PSA level 19.3. The patient elected to follow Western procedures. By a transurethral resection of the prostate (TURP), as much of the cancer was removed as possible, followed by radiation therapy.*

After the procedure, the patient's sphincter appeared to have be-come inactive and he was experiencing total urinary inconti-nence.

> *PSA factor had dropped to 7.4, which was still above the desired limit.*

PRESCRIPTION

Week 1:   *Terebinthina* 200c - daily, Plussing Method

Week 2:   *Conium* 200c - daily, Plussing Method
                 The patient's urinary control improved.

Weeks 3-8:   Same as Weeks 1-2
                 Urinary control was restored.

                 The PSA factor came down to 2.7.

Week 9:   *Conium* 200c - daily, Plussing Method

Week 10:   *Carcinosin* 200c - daily, Plussing Method

Weeks 11-40:   Same as Weeks 9-10

Months 11-15:   Same as Weeks 9-10, but in the 1M potency - alternating semimonthly, Split Dose Method

Months 16-20: Same as Weeks 9-10 - alternating monthly, Split Dose Method

> *Between Months 3 and 20, in regular, periodic rectal examinations, PSA level checks, and one CT scan of the abdomen findings were normal.*

End of intensive treatment; thereafter, only an occasional cancer nosode or constitutional remedy was prescribed.

REMARKS

> *Carcinosin* was prescribed once the urinary condition was healed and the doctor judged it time to address the original cancerous condition. (See also Remarks in Case 111.)

✦ If *postoperative urinary urgency* is due to sphincter problems, then *Staphysagria* is called for. If it is due to an infection of the bladder, then *Terebinthina* is the preferred remedy.

✦ *Anaesthesia:* At times one encounters the problem of ill effects from anaesthesia in patients who appear to be extra-sensitive to its action. Either it is difficult for them to emerge from the anaesthetic state or they exhibit some distressing reaction, such as severe nausea (with or without vomiting), persistent fear and anxiety, or a worrisome feeling of disorientation. In such cases, *Phosphorus* 30C or 200C is the best remedy, to be administered on an as-needed basis. If a patient is known to have a history of ill effects from anaesthesia, then the remedy can be administered preventatively—one dose prior to surgery instead of the final dose of *Arnica*—and then another dose as soon after surgery as possible. *Nux vomica* is another option when *Phosphorus* cannot assist.

Postsurgical Follow-up and Follow-through

✦ When a patient comes to the homoeopath after a successful operation, displays no symptoms, and all tests yield negative results, proceed as discussed in Chapter 3 (and as described in dozens of cases cited throughout the text).

✦ If the patient remains healthy, proceed to the long-term case management and recurrence prevention treatment *(described in Chapters 3 and 9)*.

✦ If the surgery was only partially successful (i.e., there has been only partial removal of the malignant mass or if the primary tumor cannot be located), if there is no major metastasis but some evidence of spread of the disease, or if the disease has metastasized in the past, then once again proceed as discussed in Chapter 3. Although there are numerous cases illustrating the general procedure, one additional example follows.

CASE 113   *February, 1995*

Female, 70 years, reported that over the past two to three months several glands were cropping up on the left side of her neck, in the cervical area—one of these in the supraclavicular area—all growing rapidly.

> *Excision biopsy and removal of the prominent glands showed them to be malignant; a CT scan and histopathology report revealed metastatic deposits in the area as secondaries, from a poorly differentiated carcinoma. No other tests could pinpoint where the primary tumor was.*

Although no definite stage could be established, this case was at least Stage II.

The woman was a typical *Silica:* mildly aloof; fairly fastidious and orderly; not self-assertive, but highly set in her ways. She was a picky eater, with an intolerance of milk; she looked emaciated, but had always been that way. In her teens, she had been diagnosed as having tuberculosis, but was fully cured after one year of treatment.

PRESCRIPTION

Week 1:   *Scrophularia nodosa* 200c - daily, Plussing Method

Week 2:   *Carcinosin* 200c - daily, Plussing Method
                 The unhealed wound where the glands had been
                 removed healed 90%, and an adjacent gland that
                 had not been removed was less indurated.

Weeks 3-6:   Same as Weeks 1-2
                 All glands in the cervical region more than 50%
                 reduced and one had almost entirely disappeared.

                 *CT scan confirmed the reduction in the size of
                 glands and showed the parenchymal infiltration
                 more than 50% resolved.*

Weeks 7-14:   Same as Weeks 1-2

                 Tests showed no change.

Weeks 15-23:   Same as Weeks 1-2, but in the 1M potency
                 The patient felt well and cheerful.

                 Tests showed not much change.

At this point, the woman grew unwilling to comply with the
Plussing Method, so the Split Dose Method was introduced.

Weeks 24-32:   *Silica* 200c† - weekly, Split Dose Method
                 The patient was stable, comfortable, and
                 asymptomatic.

                 *Tests showed that the condition remained the
                 same; no further reduction in the size of glands.
                 Still no signs of the primary
                 lesion.*

Months 9-12:   Same as Weeks 24-32, but semimonthly

Thereafter, and to this day, the patient has been receiving, periodically (usually quarterly), single doses of one of the three remedies, as her symptoms indicate. Five years later, her condition is
still stable.

REMARKS

Scrophularia nodosa opened the case because of the remedy's affinity for the glands—especially when there is a tubercular background.

Silica, the constitutional remedy, was introduced when *Scrophularia nodosa* had obviously exhausted its action. One point of note: when there is a history of pulmonary tubercular lesions, *Silica* should be prescribed only in the higher potencies, especially to the elderly. Dr. Ramakrishnan has witnessed the lower potencies open up old healed lesions, break down fibrosis, and bring about a relapse.

✦ If surgery is not successful, tumor is inoperable, and/or there is major metastasis, then proceed to the palliation methods described in Chapters 5 and 6. An example follows.

CASE 114 [p-P]   *January, 1990*

Female, 66 years, presented with an inoperable uterine cancer, Stage IV. Present symptoms were frequent urination, bladder incontinence, severe burning during micturition, pain all over the abdomen, and weakness.

> *History: Cancer of the uterus diagnosed two years previously. The mass and entire uterus were adherent to the bladder and posterior wall of pelvis— hence inoperable. The patient was treated with chemotherapy and radiation therapy.*

The woman had had bad asthma all her life and was presently on steroids. She also had several episodes of benign polyps in the colon that had been removed surgically—both symptoms pointing to *Thuja*.

PRESCRIPTION

Week 1:   *Thuja* 200c† - daily, Split Dose Method
                 Urinary symptoms slightly improved.

Week 2:	*Carcinosin* 200c - daily, Split Dose Method
Weeks 3-8:	Same as Weeks 1-2 Urinary symptoms continued to improve and abdominal pain was much less. Weakness almost gone; patient started going out shopping, etc.
Week 9:	*Thuja* 200c - once, Split Dose Method
Week 10:	*Carcinosin* 200c - once, Split Dose Method The patient was now free of bladder symptoms, and there was no more abdominal pain.
Weeks 11-20:	Same as Weeks 9-10 Energy level was maintained.
Months 5-10:	Same as Weeks 9-10 On and off severe uterine pain with profuse bleeding was controlled by *Aconite* 200c or *Magnesia phosphorica* 200c; sometimes uterine spasms required *Viburnum prunifolium* 200c—all these remedies were given ten times, at half-hour intervals, whenever needed.

The woman was relatively comfortable and active during this time. But toward the end of the tenth month, she developed severe ascites and died a few days later.

REMARKS

Today, with the Plussing Method, the woman's life would probably have been prolonged.

Needle Biopsies

A related surgical procedure is the needle biopsy of breast, bone, liver, or lymph nodes. The homoeopathic procedure to lessen the trauma is as follows:

1. The patient should be instructed to take a dose of *Bellis perennis* 200c or 30c on the day prior to a needle biopsy of the breast. The remedy

should be repeated shortly before and again soon after the procedure. Thereafter, it can be taken on an as-needed basis, for as long as there is pain.

2. For bone biopsies and harvesting of bone marrow, *Symphytum* 200C or 30C should be prescribed in the same way as *Bellis perennis*.

3. For all other needle biopsies, such as of the liver or lymph nodes, *Arnica* 200C is used in the same way as *Bellis perennis*.

Chemotherapy

Generally speaking, chemotherapy is not viewed by homoeopaths as favorably as is surgery. Especially during the later stages of cancer it is not recommended, because it weakens the vital force and undermines the body's self-healing powers, which the homoeopathic remedies try to strengthen. Moreover, the homoeopathic remedies are often antidoted by chemotherapy. As a rule, the two therapies should not be used simultaneously.

✦ Ideally, the patient should, with the cooperation and approval of his oncologist, discontinue chemotherapy as soon as possible and begin the homoeopathic treatment according to the Plussing Method.

✦ If the patient seeking homoeopathic treatment must remain on chemotherapy, but the chemotherapy is given intermittently in short-term courses, homoeopathy can be given on the days or weeks between the rounds of chemotherapy—here again, using the Plussing Method.

CASE 115   *January, 1996*

Male, 53 years, sought homoeopathic treatment for weakness, exhaustion, and emaciation following a pancreatic cancer operation. He was diagnosed as being in Stage III.

> *The removal of a mass at the head of the pancreas had been followed by chemotherapy, which completely exhausted him.*

PRESCRIPTION

Week 1:   *Ceanothus americanus* 200c - daily, Plussing
             Method

Week 2:   *Carcinosin* 200c - daily, Plussing Method
             The patient felt much better.

Weeks 3-4:   Same as Weeks 1-2
             Improvement was dramatic.

Months 2-7: Chemotherapy resumed, but in short rounds. In
             between, the patient would go on homoeopathic
             remedies using the daily, Plussing Method—until
             the next round of chemotherapy.

At the end of seven months, the patient had gained 30 lb. and was
feeling healthy. He continued the chemotherapy (in short rounds)
for a total of twelve months.

Months 8-19: Same as Weeks 1-2

The patient continues to this day on the same two remedies, but
alternating monthly, Split Dose Method. Almost five years later, he
is still doing well.

REMARKS

This case is an illustration of how homoeopathy can (if need be)
work alongside chemotherapy.

For the selection of *Ceanothus americanus,* see Chapter 2.

✦ Sometimes a patient after a mastectomy will be put on a long-
term (perhaps five-year) course of an antineoplastic/antiestrogen drug
such as tamoxifen, or a patient with multiple myeloma will be put on
methotrexate, an antimetabolite/folic acid antagonist, for an indefinite
period of time. Although this chemotherapy might to a certain extent interfere with the homoeopathic treatment, by employing the intensive
Plussing Method the patient could still benefit from the homoeopathic
medicines. And, with time, he or she may decide to discontinue the
chemotherapy.

CASE 116   *March, 1994*

Male, 55 years, presented with a collapsed vertebrae. There was much pain and discomfort.

> *Diagnosis: Multiple myeloma, Stage IV.*
> *Methotrexate was prescribed by the oncologist.*

PRESCRIPTION

Week 1:   *Hekla lava* 200C - daily, Plussing Method

Week 2:   *Carcinosin* 200C - daily, Plussing Method
             Calcarea fluorica 6X was also prescribed, to be taken three times a day for an indefinite period of time.

Weeks 3-16: Same as Weeks 1-2
             The patient's symptoms showed improvement. Pain and discomfort lessened. He decided to stop taking the methotrexate.

Months 5-8: Same as Weeks 1-2, but in the 1M potency
             The patient continued to improve.

             CT scan showed arrest of disease, which was considered to be a good report.

Months 9-18: *Hekla lava* 1M and *Carcinosin* 1M - alternating monthly, Split Dose Method

             Quarterly CT scans of spine continued to show that there was no further deterioration of the condition.

The patient continued with daily doses of the *Calcarea fluorica* cell salt. He also continued with the regimen of Months 9-18. After three years, the cancer metastasized to the skull and he died shortly thereafter.

REMARKS

Although the patient died after four and a half years, given the type and stage of his cancer, he did remarkably well. (See also Case 65.)

✦ Homoeopathy has likewise proven invaluable when there has been metastasis after chemotherapy—whether the chemotherapy followed surgery or not (see Cases 36, 37, and many others).

✦ Finally, there are several homoeopathic remedies that have proven of assistance to patients who are undergoing or have undergone a course of chemotherapy and are suffering from its side effects.

✦ *Cadmium sulphuratum* is the preferred remedy for the weakness, nausea, and vomiting during or following chemotherapy.

CASE 117   *April, 1993*

Male, 43 years, presented with weakness and prostration after being operated on for a huge mass on the head of the pancreas, followed by intensive chemotherapy. This left the patient totally exhausted; he wanted to lie still—and not be touched or moved. He was diagnosed as being in Stage III.

> *The mass operated on had been pressing on the duodenum and bile duct, and only two-thirds of it could be removed.*

PRESCRIPTION

Week 1:   *Cadmium sulphuratum* 200c - daily, Plussing Method

Week 2:   *Carcinosin* 200c - daily, Plussing Method
                 The patient's prostration had lessened somewhat.

Weeks 3-16:   Same as Weeks 1-2
                 The patient continued slowly to improve.

Weeks 17-20:   Same as Weeks 1-2, but in the 1M potency
The patient was now physically much improved, but began exhibiting symptoms of fear and anxiety. Also, his innate fastidiousness began to reassert itself.

Weeks 21-22:   *Arsenicum album* 200c† (for the above symptoms) - daily, Plussing Method
The patient's attitude improved dramatically and he was feeling almost normal.

Week 23:   *Carcinosin* 200c - daily, Plussing Method

Weeks 24-48:   Same as Weeks 21-23
The patient felt well, physically and mentally.

For six years, now, the patient has been receiving *Arsenicum album* 200c and *Carcinosin* 200c, alternating monthly, Split Dose Method.

REMARKS

For the prescription of *Cadmium sulphuratum,* see Chapters 2 and 6; also, Case 80.

✦ If *Cadmium sulphuratum* is not effective, the other reliable standbys for discomfort associated with chemotherapy are *Arsenicum album* and *Nux vomica;* also, *Ipecacuanha* for uncontrolled vomiting.

Radiation Therapy

Just as homoeopaths generally do not recommend chemotherapy, so, except for pain relief during the terminal stages of cancer, they generally do not recommend radiation therapy. Far more comfort and relief are obtained from the homoeopathic remedies *(see Chapter 5).* As a rule, homoeopathic treatment should *not* be given throughout the duration of radiation therapy, but it can be commenced as soon as the course is terminated; it can also be given when there has been metastasis after radiation (see Cases 37, 46, and others).

✦ For the patient who suffers from depletion and/or external or internal burning sensations after radiation therapy, the best remedy is often *Radium bromide,* to be administered in the 200C potency until symptoms are better.

CASE 118   *September, 1998*

Female, 41 years, reported with severe burns from radiation; also a breast ulcer that would not heal, with much burning pain.

> *History: A cancer of the right breast, Stage III, had recently been operated on, followed by chemotherapy and radiation. The radiation produced extensive burns, and the patient turned to homoeopathy.*

PRESCRIPTION

Week 1:   *Radium bromide* 200C - daily, Plussing Method

Week 2:   *Carcinosin* 200C - daily, Plussing Method
                 Also, *Arsenicum iodatum* 6X, twice a day for the local infection.
                 The patient felt much better.

Weeks 3-12:   Same as Weeks 1-2
                 The patient continued to heal very nicely.

Weeks 13-24:   Same as Weeks 1-2
                 Burns entirely healed.

> *Routine tests had picked up two suspicious spots in the pelvic bone.*

Week 25:   *Hekla lava* 200C - daily, Plussing Method

Week 26:   *Carcinosin* 200C - daily, Plussing Method

Weeks 27-40:   Same as Weeks 25-26

> *After this treatment, everything showed clear.*

Months 11-15: Same as Weeks 25-26, but alternating weekly, Split
Dose Method

Tests continued to show everything clear.

Thereafter, and to this day, the woman has received doses of her
constitutional remedy *Natrum muriaticum* 1M (see Case 90 for
personality traits) and *Carcinosin* 1M, alternating monthly, Split
Dose Method.

✦ If the patient obtains no relief or shows no improvement from
Radium bromide, the second best remedies are potentized *X-ray* or *Can-
tharis.*

✦ Even if a patient displays no apparent ill effects from radiotherapy, one dose of potentized *X-ray* 200C for three days in succession is advisable, so as to clean out the X-ray residues and counteract possible side
effects.

✦ At any point during or after radiotherapy, the patient can apply
Urtica urens ointment to the burnt area, on an as-needed basis. It has repeatedly proven remarkably effective.

One final and completely separate point to bear in mind is that the
symptomatic or clinical condition of a patient is not always reflected by
Western procedures and tests. The following case offers an example of this
discrepancy—and of how a patient under systematic homoeopathic treatment can live long and comfortably with a cancer, even if the pathological
picture does not change.

CASE 119   *June, 1993*

Female, 52 years, presented with metastasis in lungs, bladder, and
several mesenteric glands. She was experiencing pain in the abdomen, blood in the urine, and bloody expectorations. She was
diagnosed as being in Stage III.

History: In May, 1992, patient had been operated on for ovarian cancer, followed by radiation therapy.

PRESCRIPTION

Week 1: *Aurum muriaticum natronatum* 200c - daily, Plussing Method

Week 2: *Carcinosin* 200c - daily, Plussing Method

Weeks 3-12: Same as Weeks 1-2
Concomitantly, *Arsenicum iodatum* 6x was used all along for the infections the patient suffered, whether in bladder, lungs, or elsewhere.

CT scan showed no change, but also no progress of the disease.

Months 4-10: Same as Weeks 1-2, but in the 1M potency
The patient was doing well. No hemoptysis, hematuria, dysuria; no pain in abdomen; gaining a little weight.

Periodic scans showed no change, but also no deterioration of condition.

Months 11-16: Same as Months 4-10, but in the 10M potency

For two full years, the woman remained on the same two remedies in the 10M potency, alternating monthly, Split Dose Method. Thereafter, she would receive these two remedies, alternating quarterly. Seven years later, a CT scan showed no change whatsoever, but the patient's condition has remained clinically stable and she feels strong and cheerful.

REMARKS

The value of *Aurum muriaticum natronatum* in cancers of the female reproductive system (in this case, the site of the primary cancer) was discussed in Chapter 2.

Additional instances of the discrepancy between pathology reports and the patient's clinical condition are found in Cases 19, 24, 102, 113, and several others.

Chapter 9

Homoeopathy in Cancer Prevention

A unique feature of homoeopathy is the remedies' *preventive* roles in different types of ailments and illnesses. For instance, *Tuberculinum,* prescribed in the autumn, can avert winter coughs or other respiratory tract infections in a patient inherently susceptible to these; periodic doses of *Gelsemium* have helped stave off influenza; a course of *Rhus toxicodendron* can desensitize a patient to poison ivy; and so forth. In the "prevention" of cancer, the results, to be sure, are impossible to gauge. After all, there is no telling who will succumb to the disease and who will not—and when or whether it will recur after a "cure." But patients at greater risk due to a strong family history of cancer or from having had cancer might well be strengthened against the likelihood of developing the disease by certain homoeopathic procedures.

Counteracting a Family History of Cancer

Carcinosin, as was noted earlier, is the preferred nosode if there is a family history of cancer. In the patient exhibiting no signs of the disease, a single dose of the remedy, in the 200c potency, three or four times a year, is an advisable preventive measure. If the patient is under regular homoeopathic treatment, *Carcinosin* 1M can be prescribed twice a year in between the constitutional remedies.

Prevention of Recurrence

Patients who are experiencing a recurrence require a longer course of treatment to reduce the chances of further recurrence. Many such cases have been encountered earlier in this book, but an additional one follows.

CASE 120   *July, 1995*

Female, 39 years, presented with a recurrence after an operation for cancer of the right ovary, performed a year earlier.

> *History: In summer, 1994, tests showed adenocarcinoma of the ovary, Stage IIc, which was operated on, then followed up with chemotherapy.*

The woman was pretty, with large, sparkling eyes; by nature high-strung and of artistic temperament; friendly and constantly seeking assurance of others' affection. She complained of pain in the right iliac fossa (the area of recurrence), also of occasionally experiencing a white or bloody vaginal discharge, and all her life she had been prone to heavy nosebleeds—characteristics and symptoms all suggestive of *Phosphorus*.

PRESCRIPTION

Week 1:   *Phosphorus* 200c† - daily, Plussing Method

Week 2:   *Carcinosin* 200c - daily, Plussing Method

Weeks 3-8:   Same as Weeks 1-2
                The patient was comfortable.

> *CT scan showed absolutely no change in the size of the mass.*

Week 9:   *Aurum muriaticum natronatum* 200c - daily, Plussing Method

Week 10:   *Carcinosin* 200c - daily, Plussing Method

Weeks 11-20:   Same as Weeks 9-10
                The patient put on weight; weakness and anemia were considerably reduced.

Physical examination and CT scan showed reduction of the mass.

Months 6-9:   Same as Weeks 9-10

Physical examination and CT scan showed further reduction of mass.

Months 10-15: Same as Weeks 9-10, but in the 1M potency

Physical examination and CT scan showed still further reduction of the mass.

Months 15-24: Same as Weeks 9-10, but in the 10M potency

At 18 months, CT scan showed the mass had completely disappeared; less-frequent scans thereafter continued to show everything clear.

After two years, the woman was taken off the Plussing Method and moved on to her constitutional remedy, *Phosphorus* 1M, alternating semimonthly with *Carcinosin* 1M. This regimen continues to date.

Blood tumor markers and results of CT scans have been absolutely normal.

REMARKS

Although *Phosphorus* fit the patient's overall picture well and has also proven of use in the treatment of ovarian cancer, the results were not good enough to justify continuing with it—and the greater "organ-specific" remedy was resorted to.

When *Aurum muriaticum natronatum* had exhausted its action, Dr. Ramakrishnan could return to the constitutional remedy, but continued with the cancer nosode as well.

The Schuessler Tissue/Cell Salts

The use of *Schuessler Tissue/Cell Salts* in maintenance treatment is optional. A number of patients derive comfort from taking them for one or two years, even after they are, to all appearances, free of the disease (or once the cancer has stabilized). Although, here again, it is difficult to gauge the Cell Salts's preventive role, often they have been found to be effective in relief of specific groups of symptoms, both during treatment of the disease and in long-term maintenance.

> *Calcarea fluorica* is often employed in the maintenance of bone cancer;
> *Ferrum phosphoricum* for blood cancer;
> *Natrum muriaticum* in cancer of the skin;
> *Natrum phosphoricum* in cancer of the bladder;
> *Natrum sulphuricum* for cancer of the pancreas; and
> *Silica* in cancer that affects the periosteum.

The most common way of prescribing the Cell Salts for maintenance is in the 6x potency, but the 6c or 3x or 3c or 12x (and other low potencies) are also employed. The length of time they are taken varies according to the type and severity of the cancer; in Dr. Ramakrishnan's experience, two years is the usual length of time—although they can be taken indefinitely. The following case exemplifies the long-term use of a cell salt (see also Case 116).

CASE 121 [p-P]   *June, 1991*

Male, 40 years, presented with a mass in the right temporal region. He was rapidly losing weight, was tired, had no appetite, but fortunately was not experiencing much pain.

> *MRI revealed a conical space-occupying lesion next to the right orbit. The biopsy performed at the right temporal region revealed a round cell undifferentiated malignant tumor, Stage III. X-ray evaluation of the chest and spine revealed deposits in cervical ribs, clavicles, and vertebrae. Differential*

diagnosis: (1) metastasis, (2) lachrymal duct tumor, (3) lymphoma. The patient opted for only homoeopathic treatment.

The patient was dazed, not very responsive, and was either too hot or too cold. No other symptoms could be elicited.

PRESCRIPTION

Weeks 1-2: *Symphytum* 30c - daily, Split Dose Method
The patient was slightly better; more alert.

Weeks 3-8: *Symphytum* 200c - daily, Split Dose Method
The patient continued slightly better all round.

Weeks 9-10: *Symphytum* 10M - daily, Split Dose Method
Only very slight improvement; hence the need to look for another remedy.

Weeks 11-12: *Hekla lava* 200c - daily, Split Dose Method
Swelling subsided substantially. General condition better.

Month 4: Same as Weeks 11-12
Mass almost gone.

Month 5: Same as Weeks 11-12
The patient was free of symptoms, with swelling completely subsided.

All this time, the patient was unwilling to undergo any more MRIs, scans, or x-ray evaluations, so what happened to the brain lesion or the secondaries was not known.

Months 6-12: Same as Weeks 11-12
The patient remained entirely symptom free.

Thereafter, the patient received *Calcarea fluorica* 6x, twice a day, and continues to take it until the present day. He moved, but stays in touch regularly with Dr. Ramakrishnan to report that he continues to do well.

> *The patient continues to be uncooperative and not to go for anymore x-ray evaluations, so what happened to the primary lesion or the secondaries is still not known.*

REMARKS

In this case, the organ-specific remedy, *Hekla lava,* needed no assistance from a cancer nosode or constitutional remedy to effect its healing. But another "specific" for the bones, the *Calcarea fluorica* Cell Salt, has, over the years, maintained the good work of *Hekla lava.*

Remedies other than cell salts can also be used in low potency for maintenance and prevention of recurrences. For instance, *Sabal serrulata* 6x, two or three times a day, might stave off a recurrence of prostate cancer and, in Case 64, *Iodum* 6x was used to prevent a recurrence of Hodgkin's lymphoma.

Prevention in Precancerous Conditions

In this category one is no longer dealing with unknowables but with clearly documented evidence of the homoeopathic remedies' capacity to arrest the spread of the disease and even to reverse pathology. Among the most commonly encountered precancerous conditions are those of the oral cavity, prostate, cervix, and the skin. The most common way of prescribing for these conditions is the appropriate remedy in the 200c potency, daily, weekly, or semimonthly, *using the Split Dose Method.* Continue this method for several months—at which point there should be a visible and/or measurable improvement.

Precancer of the Oral Cavity

Leukoplakia, or white patches on the tongue or inside of the cheek (sometimes occurring in tobacco-chewers or heavy smokers), can be considered a precancerous condition. Ninety percent of these cases call for *Aurum muriaticum.*

CASE 122   *January, 1995*

Male, 53 years, a tobacco-chewer, presented with leukoplakia of both cheeks.

PRESCRIPTION

Month 1:   *Aurum muriaticum* 200c - semimonthly, Split Dose Method
               Tobacco-chewing was discontinued.

Months 2-3:   Same as Month 1
               Leukoplakia 75% healed.

Months 4-6:   Same as Month 1
               Condition totally cleared.

End of treatment. The patient has remained completely healthy for more than five years now.

Precancer of the Prostate

As discussed in Chapter 2, when the PSA count is marginally elevated (between 4 and 7), *Thuja* is generally the preferred remedy. If the count is 7 or higher, *Conium* generally takes precedence.

CASE 123   *November, 1996*

Male, 53 years, presented with an elevated PSA count of 14.

                    Digital rectal examination and CT scan yielded normal results.

PRESCRIPTION

Month 1:   *Conium* 200c - semimonthly, Split Dose Method

Month 2:   *Carcinosin* 200c - semimonthly, Split Dose Method

Months 3-5:   Same as Months 1-2

                    PSA count came down to 9.

Months 6-12:   Same as Months 1-2

> *PSA count came down to 2.5.*

Months 13-24: Same as Months 1-2

> *The PSA count came down to 0.5—and has remained at this level ever since.*

No further treatment.

REMARKS

Carcinosin was selected over *Scirrhinum* because the patient's condition was *precancerous*—for which the former nosode is more frequently employed.

The above is the classical way of treating a precancerous state of the prostate with elevated PSA count. The following case exemplifies how one may need to find an alternative way.

CASE 124   *January, 1996*

Male, 66 years, presented with an elevated PSA count of 12. There were no other symptoms; and a routine checkup showed everything normal.

PRESCRIPTION

Week 1:   *Conium* 200c - daily, Split Dose Method

Week 2:   *Carcinosin* 200c - daily, Split Dose Method

Weeks 3-8:   Same as Weeks 1-2

> *PSA count was 11.5.*

Month 3:   Same as Weeks 1-2

> *No change in PSA count.*

Months 4-5:   *Sabal serrulata* 200c - daily, Split Dose Method

> *PSA count was down to 7.*

Months 6-7: *Sabal serrulata* 1M - weekly, Split Dose Method

> *PSA count was 3.1.*

Months 8-12: *Sabal serrulata* 1M - semimonthly, Split Dose Method

> *PSA count fluctuated between 2.1 and 3.1.*

End of treatment. The patient continues to do well to date.

> *PSA count continues to fluctuate between 2.1 and 3.1.*

REMARKS

Dr. Ramakrishnan did not feel the need to return to the use of a cancer nosode, since the patient was responding so well to *Sabal serrulata*.

Precancer of the Cervix

CASE 125   *August, 1995*

Female, 37 years, presented with a Papanicolaou (Pap) smear result that was positive for cancer.

> *History: In 1994, a gynecological exam for patient's excessive leucorrhea revealed an erosion of the cervix. The biopsy result was negative for cancer; hence only cauterization was performed. A routine examination in 1995 showed the cervix healthy, the uterus normal, but the Pap smear continued to yield positive results.*

PRESCRIPTION

Month 1: *Aurum muriaticum natronatum* 200c - semimonthly, Split Dose Method

Month 2: *Carcinosin* 200c - semimonthly, Split Dose Method

Months 3-6:   Same as Months 1-2

> *Pap smear test was negative; and repeated tests over the years have yielded negative results.*

REMARKS

This is just one of numerous similar cases. The above combination of remedies for a positive Pap smear is the one Dr. Ramakrishnan always starts with, and only moves on to one of the other remedies that have been found to be useful for positive Pap smears—*Sepia, Pulsatilla, Medorrhinum*—if the first combination does not work. These last remedies should be prescribed alternately with *Carcinosin,* in a manner similar to the case above.

Lichen Planus and Other Precancerous Skin Conditions

These respond well to homoeopathy. Among the best remedies are *Arsenicum album, Arsenicum iodatum,* and *Calcarea arsenica.*

CASE 126   *April, 1998*

Female, 36 years, presented with a severe case of lichen planus. Her symptoms were: lesions distributed all over, with the skin peeling, then ulcerating and forming a black scab: intense burning, relieved by warm applications. All this was typical of *Arsenicum album.*

PRESCRIPTION

Months 1-4:   *Arsenicum album* 200C - semimonthly, Split Dose Method

> *The patient was monitored once a month and by the end of four months, lesions cleared 50%.*

Months 5-8:   Same as Weeks 1-16, but in the 1M potency

> *Full recovery. All lesions cleared.*

Thereafter, and for the next year, *Arsenicum album* 1M was prescribed monthly, Split Dose Method. The woman reports in regularly and is doing well.

REMARKS

Although by no means does every lichen planus turn into a cancerous condition, it can be a predisposing factor and hence requires care and attention.

In its preventive role, homoeopathy is inevitably limited. True cancer prevention lies in a larger—the global—realm. In her groundbreaking book, *Silent Spring*, Rachel Carson made a strong argument that the basic issue is the pollution of the environment with chemicals and radiation, which then adversely affects the delicate balance of the human ecology, leaving it more vulnerable to malignancy ("Human exposures to cancer-producing agents are uncontrolled and they are multiple"). But although offering no magic "preventive pill" as protection against cancer, homoeopathy does often play a significant role in strengthening the system—in this way, perhaps, making the human constitution more resistant to environmental contaminants.

Concluding Remarks

The homoeopathic discipline consists of a highly specific method of administering its medicines—and, as we have seen in the foregoing chapters, in cases of cancer an even stricter methodology has been found to be necessary to obtain the best results. But since individualization always remains a primary tenet in homoeopathic prescribing, assessing when to change remedies, move on to higher potencies, or alter procedures of prescribing cannot be reduced to hard and fast rules. These issues every homoeopath must decide for himself. Therefore, the case examples encountered in these pages do not establish definitive formulas. Rather, presented in such a form as to allow them to speak largely for themselves, they are offered as guiding models in prescribing for the different types of cancer.

The objective of this book is to empower. Without underestimating the many difficulties entailed in the treatment of cancer (the hard work, the strong commitment, and the patience to persevere), the sheer volume of these cases, illustrating Dr. Ramakrishnan's often successful method and reflecting his vast experience, is intended to encourage the prescriber to try administering the homoeopathic remedies in conjunction with the appropriate (minimally invasive) Western medical procedures. In this way, patients suffering from cancer can be given additional hope and healing assistance.

Appendix
Frequently Asked Questions— and Answers

1 Q: *How long will the treatment take?*

A: Eighteen months at least. The length of time depends on the type and the stage of the cancer *(see Chapter 3)*.

2 Q: *How rigid is the Plussing Method? Must the timing of "fifteen minutes between each dose" be exact?*

A: Even though occasional lapses will not jeopardize the treatment, the importance of adhering to the procedure described in this book (especially until the tumor is under control) cannot be overemphasized. If strict adherence to the fifteen-minute intervals is impossible, it is preferable to shorten the time between the ten doses rather than to omit a dose (although there is no harm if one dose in the midst of the ten is slightly late).

3 Q: *Can one split up the ten doses and take them during different times of the day, say half in the morning and half in the evening?*

A: No. The ten doses should be taken during the one block of time.

4 Q: *Can any food or drink be partaken of during the two and a half hours of taking the medicine?*

A: No food should be eaten; but very ill patients may have weak tea or juice during the "plussing" time, between the doses. Water is permissible at all times.

5   Q: *What happens if, due to circumstances beyond a patient's control, he skips a day—or even two?*

   A: It need not be crucial. But the patient should get back on schedule immediately—and should not make a habit of skipping even *one* day. Skipping the remedies happens mostly during hospitalization, so it is essential to have a committed caretaker overseeing the plussing regimen. The only legitimate days the remedies can be skipped are those on which chemotherapy or radiation therapy is administered.

6   Q: *Does one ever get a rest from the Plussing Method?*

   A: Occasionally Dr. Ramakrishnan judges it is safe for a patient to take a short vacation (maybe a week or two) from the strict medicinal regimen—but this is not timed to personal convenience. This occurs only when the patient is no longer in a critical condition, the disease has stabilized, and the tumor is under control (see Case 56). Otherwise, no—there is no respite from the regimen until the patient is deemed well enough to progress to more infrequent dosages *(see Chapter 3).*

7   Q: *Is any time of the day best for the Plussing Method? And must this be constant?*

   A: The patient can choose anytime at his own convenience—and he can vary the time from day to day, as his schedule requires.

8   Q: *In the Plussing Method, does one add fresh medicine to the water every day?*

   A: No. Only put medicine in water on the first day of the weekly prescription *(see Chapter 1).*

9   Q: *Does one save the teaspoon of the plussed remedy that remains at the end of the week for the next round of the same, starting a week later?*

   A: No. At the end of the week, before moving on to the second remedy, one finishes off the week's supply. When returning to the first remedy, one week later, one starts with a fresh preparation.

10   Q: *Where and how does one keep the "plussed" medicine?*

A: Keep in a closed glass jar in a cool place, preferably in the refrigerator. If traveling, or on vacation, do not be overly concerned if medicine is not kept refrigerated, or even cool. It will still work. And for convenience, one can temporarily resort to a plastic container.

But note that each remedy must have its own glass jar. Even after washing it, do not use the same jar for different remedies or for different potencies of the same remedy.

11   Q: *What happens to the Plussing Method when a patient requires some other homoeopathic remedy for an acute or specific condition that must be addressed?*

A: This issue is discussed in detail in Chapter 7. But to summarize, one continues with the "plussed" remedies throughout, working around them with the "acute" remedy.

12   Q: *What about allopathic medicines? Are they incompatible and will they interfere with the homoeopathic remedies?*

A: Not always. It is, of course, preferable to take as little allopathic medication as possible, although certain medications (such as for heart, thyroid, seizures, or diabetes) must be continued. These are worked round the "plussing" procedure (i.e., some time is allowed to elapse between).

Then there are the narcotics and painkillers. In the earlier stages, narcotics can interfere with the effectiveness of homoeopathic treatment by disguising guiding symptoms or overpowering the action of the remedies. But in the later stage, when they are so often indispensable, they can work in tandem with homoeopathy (see p. 171).

13   Q: *What about the timing of the Split Dose—how precise must it be?*

A: The four parts of the single split remedy can be spread out during the day at a patient's convenience, as long as they are taken at least half an hour before or after meals or brushing the teeth—and as far apart from other medication as possible.

14   Q: *The remedies come prepared in different shapes and sizes. How is a patient to know* exactly *how much to take in dry form or how much to put in water for plussing?*

A: The patient need not disquiet himself over the exact amount of medicated globules/pellets/granules/grains to take. *Quantity does not matter in homoeopathy.* Taking three pellets or thirty is the same. A standard dose when using the Plussing Method is three pellets or globules or the number of granules or grains amounting roughly to the size of a pea. *Most important is not to agonize over this question.*

15   Q: *Do the Schuessler Tissue/Cell Salts interfere with the Ramakrishnan Method? For how long should they be taken?*

A: Since the Schuessler Cell Salts often play an integral role in the process of healing, during the more intensive Plussing Method treatment, they should be taken only as prescribed by the practitioner. Once the case is stabilized, however, or in long-term maintenance, they can be used regularly, if the patient so wishes and for as long as he wishes. For more on this subject, see Chapter 9.

16   Q: *In his treatment of cancer, does Dr. Ramakrishnan ever employ a potentized preparation made of the matter extracted from a patient's own malignant tumor?*

A: Dr. Ramakrishnan does not use such preparations himself—insofar as they have not been "proven" (see footnote, p. 7) and are based on the principle of "sameness" and not, strictly speaking, on the homoeopathic "similarity"; also he has not seen enough good results to use this method himself. It does not mean, however, that this form of "isopathic" treatment could not be administered by the Plussing Method, if some practitioner chooses to do so.

17   Q: *Can other nosodes be employed using the Plussing Method, apart from the two cancer ones?*

A: Because, in cancer cases, Dr. Ramakrishnan has obtained the best results with *Carcinosin* and *Scirrhinum,* today he employs these two nosodes almost exclusively. However, occasionally, when the symptoms dictate, he will use another nosode (Plussing Method)—as in Case 95, where *Tuberculinum* was prescribed.

18   Q: *What is the optimum frequency of visits to the doctor or of telephone follow-ups during treatment?*

A: Until the disease is under control, monthly visits or phone follow-ups are essential. After stabilization of the cancer, three to six visits a year (in person or by phone) are strongly recommended, these to continue for at least two years. In Stage IV of the disease, the more frequent changes in prescription, potency, or remedy repetition may well require closer supervision.

19   Q: *Can the Plussing Method be applied to other illnesses?*

A: No—the Plussing Method, as developed and employed by Dr. Ramakrishnan, is reserved for cancer only *(see final paragraph in Chapter 3)*.

20   Q: *How does the Ramakrishnan Method work in conjunction with other alternative therapies?*

A: Although this question, and the two that follow it, do not lie strictly within the jurisdiction of this book, because a number of patients seeking homoeopathic assistance have undergone or are undergoing some alternative therapy, it will be briefly addressed. Therapies such as acupuncture, chiropractic, Reiki, shiatsu, or other forms of hands-on or body therapy (all of which work along the same lines as homoeopathy, trying to stimulate the life force and the body's self-healing powers) can be of assistance working in conjunction with homoeopathy—whether bringing relief from pain, enhancing the quality of life, or encouraging the process of healing.

Although Chinese herbs can be a highly effective cancer therapy in their own right, to avoid confusion, Dr. Ramakrishnan prefers that two different healing stimuli not be used simultaneously during the more intense period of homoeopathic treatment.

Sometimes, however, and especially once the patient is no longer in a critical condition, Chinese herbs can be used in alternation with the homoeopathic remedies with good effect.

Tibetan medicines are somewhat different. Acting more along the line of supplements, these efficacious herbs and minerals can be taken in conjunction with homoeopathy.

Dr. Ramakrishnan does not object to the use of anthroposophic *Iscador®* (mistletoe) during the course of his treatment, because he has not found it to interfere.

The use of Western herbs, magnets, and machines that change the body's electromagnetic field are *not* recommended, because Dr. Ramakrishnan feels these therapies can interfere with his treatment.

21   Q: *Does the Ramakrishnan Method demand that the patient follow any special diet during the course of treatment?*

A: No particular diet is recommended, nor do patients have to follow any stringent dietary rules. Not because Dr. Ramakrishnan does not consider this subject important, but because he tries to disrupt normal life and eating habits as little as possible. He also recognizes that nutrition is a highly individual subject (literally, "one man's meat is another man's poison"), that the needs of the body vary during the different stages of the cancer, and that each patient must find his own most comfortable and beneficial diet.

From Hahnemann on down, however, homoeopaths have always stressed the importance of a good and balanced diet. This entails plenty of fresh vegetables and fruit, beans and *sprouted* or *whole* grains, and the corollary minimizing of sugar and highly processed foods. Moderation and common sense play a significant role in nutrition—although due to the hormone and other additives in meat and dairy products, a number of homoeopaths will recommend a largely vegetarian diet (especially with an avoidance of dairy and red meat). Also, in view of the high use of pesticides and other chemicals in farming, organically grown produce is always preferable.

Perhaps the one constant guiding rule here is, "Try to eat as healthfully as you know how, in order to give the homoeopathic remedies the best chance you can."

22 Q: *What about vitamins and supplements—do they interfere with homoeopathic treatment?*

A: Vitamins and supplements do not interfere with the homoeopathic remedies, provided the two are not taken at the same time and at least one hour is allowed to elapse in between. And certain vitamins, such as the "anti-oxidants" (which include vitamins A, certain Bs, C, E, selenium, zinc, and other minerals) or such a supplement as coenzyme Q10 (produced by the liver in the healthy, but often found to be insufficient in patients with metastatic cancer) have proven of value.

23 Q: *Can the patient drink any coffee or alcohol?*

A: Opinion varies as to this. Some doctors, including Dr. Ramakrishnan, do not consider occasional and very moderate partaking of these substances to be harmful, except when there is liver involvement. Others feel strongly that coffee is both harmful to the nervous system and interferes with the remedies—and that alcohol, like all sugars, feeds the cancer cells. Ultimately, the question boils down to an individual's susceptibility to, and particular tolerance of, these substances.

24 Q: *Does the Ramakrishnan Method (and homoeopathy in general) require any particular change in lifestyle in a cancer patient?*

A: Nothing in particular. Here again, the patient is encouraged to pursue as normal, fulfilling, and individually comfortable a lifestyle as he can. However, believing that in disease, mind, body, and spirit are interrelated, homoeopathy never loses sight of the emotional state and psychological factors in the process of healing. Hahnemann himself wrote in his *Chronic Diseases*. "By far the most frequent aggravations of chronic ailments are caused by grief and vexation. . . . Uninterrupted grief and vexation [such as] an unhappy marriage or a remorseful conscience . . . develop into chronic sufferings more certainly and more frequently than all other injurious influences operating on the human organism in an average human life."

Although this strong statement oversimplifies a highly complex question in which hereditary and environmental factors are also involved *(see Chapter 9)*, unhealthy life conditions, such as too high-powered a business schedule, a difficult family situation, or an unhealthy mental state (consuming worries or chronic discontent) may well contribute to the disease. Conversely, an attempt to alter stressful circumstances or cultivate a healthier state of mind can assist in the healing.

Glossary of Medicines Mentioned in the Text and Their Common Names*

MEDICINE	COMMON NAME
Aconitum napellus (Aconite)	Monkshood
Aethusa cynapium	Fool's parsley
Aloe	Socotrine aloes
Apis mellifica (Apis)	Honeybee
Argentum nitricum	Silver nitrate
Arnica	Leopard's bane
Arsenicum album	Arsenic trioxide
Arsenicum bromatum	Arsenic bromide
Arsenicum iodatum	Arsenic iodide
Aurum iodatum	Aurum iodide
Aurum metallicum	Metallic gold
Aurum muriaticum	Aurum muriate
Aurum muriaticum natronatum	Sodium chloroaurate
Baryta carbonica	Baryta carbonate
Baryta iodata	Baryta iodide
Bellis perennis	Daisy

*When purchasing any of these remedies, make certain that they are potentized *homoeopathic* preparations. Herbal preparations or supplement pill form will not serve for the method described in this book.

MEDICINE	COMMON NAME
Cadmium sulphuratum	Cadmic sulphate
Calcarea arsenica	Calcium arsenite
Calcarea carbonica	Calcium carbonate
Calcarea fluorica	Calcium fluoride
Cantharis	Spanish fly
Carbo vegetabilis	Vegetable charcoal
Carcinosin	Nosode
Causticum	Hahnemann's tinctura acris sine kali
Ceanothus americanus	New Jersey tea
Chelidonium majus (Chelidonium)	Celandine
Cinchona officinalis (China)	Peruvian bark
Colocynthis	Bitter cucumber
Conium	Poison hemlock
Euphorbium	Spurge
Ferrum phosphoricum	Iron phosphate
Gelsemium	Yellow jasmine
Graphites	Black lead
Hekla lava	Lava scoriae from Mt. Hecla
Hydrastis	Goldenseal
Hypericum	St. John's wort
Iodum	Iodine
Ipecacuanha	Ipecac root
Kali bichromicum	Potash bichromate
Kali carbonicum	Carbonate of potassium
Lachesis	Venom of the bushmaster or surucucu
Lapis albus	Silico-fluoride of calcium
Lilium tigrinum	Tiger lily
Lycopodium	Club moss

MEDICINE	COMMON NAME
Magnesia phosphorica	Magnesium phosphate
Medorrhinum	Nosode
Mercurius solubilis	Hahnemann's soluble mercury
Natrum muriaticum	Sodium chloride
Natrum phosphoricum	Sodium phosphate
Natrum sulphuricum	Sodium sulphate
Nitricum acidum	Nitric acid
Nux vomica	Poison nut
Opium	Dried latex of poppy
Ornithogalum umbellatum	Star of Bethlehem
Oxalicum acidum	Sorrel acid
Phosphorus	Phosphorus
Phytolacca	Poke root
Plumbum iodatum	Lead iodide
Plumbum metallicum	Lead
Pulsatilla nigricans (Pulsatilla)	Windflower
Pyrogenium	Artificial sepsin
Radium	Radium bromide
Rhus toxicodendron	Poison ivy
Sabal serrulata	Saw palmetto
Sanguinaria	Bloodroot
Scirrhinum	Nosode
Scrophularia nodosa	Knotted figwort
Selenium	The element selenium
Sepia	Ink of the cuttlefish
Silica	Pure flint
Spongia tosta (Spongia)	Roasted sponge
Staphysagria	Stavesacre
Strontia	Carbonate of strontia
Sulphur	Sublimated sulphur
Symphytum	Comfrey

MEDICINE	COMMON NAME
Terebinthina	Turpentine
Thuja occidentalis (Thuja)	Arbor vitae
Tuberculinum bovinum	Nosode
Urtica urens	Stinging nettle
Viburnum prunifolium	Black haw
X-ray	Potentized x-ray
Zincum sulphuricum	Zinc sulphate

Bibliography of Works Cited

Boericke, William. *Materia Medica with Repertory*. New Delhi: B. Jain Publishers (n.d.).

Cancer Manual. American Cancer Society. Latest edition.

Carson, Rachel. *Silent Spring*. Boston: Houghton Mifflin, 1962.

Coulter, Catherine R.. *Nature and Human Personality: Homoeopathic Archetypes*. Berkeley Springs, West Virginia: Ninth House Publishing [originally published 2000], current edition 2002.

Coulter, Catherine R. *Portraits of Homoeopathic Medicines: Psychophysical Analyses of Selected Constitutional Types*. vols. 1, 2, and 3. Berkeley Springs, West Virginia: Ninth House Publishing [originally published 1985, 1988, and 1998 respectively], current edition 2002.

Foubister, Donald M. The *Carcinosin* Drug Picture. *The British Homoeopathic Journal*, vol. 47, no. 3. July, 1958.

Hahnemann, Samuel. *The Chronic Diseases*, vol. 1. New Delhi: B. Jain Publishers (n.d.).

Hahnemann, Samuel. *The Organon of Medicine*. Translated by R.E. Dudgeon. New Delhi: B. Jain Publishers (n.d.).

Kent, James Tyler. *Lectures on Homoeopathic Materia Medica*. New Delhi: Jain Publishing Co., 1972.

Kent, James Tyler. *General Repertory of the Homoeopathic Materia Medica*. Any one of many editions.

Tyler, Margaret. *Homoeopathic Drug Pictures*. Sussex: Health Science Press, 1970.

Index

---

*Carcinosin is used so frequently that there is no need to list every reference to this remedy.

---

*Scirrhinum is used so frequently that there is no need to list every reference to this remedy.